UNBECOMING A NURSE

BYPASSING THE HIDDEN
CHEMICAL DEPENDENCY
TRAP

by Paula Davies Scimeca, RN, MS

Library of Congress Control Number 2008910160

ISBN 978-0-9821904-0-1

Dedication

To all the nurses who have ever rendered care to others.

To those who have succumbed to the chemical dependency trap, as well as those who have escaped, by narrow margin or with room to spare.

But most especially to those who have lost their lives, and the very many people they have left behind.

Acknowledgments

I would like to thank my husband, Thomas, for his unfailing support. Without his financial backing, this book would have gone unwritten. Thank you for encouraging in me what you may never fully understand. Your devotion to this project has furthered chemical dependency awareness and prevention efforts in my beloved profession, nursing.

Words fail to express my deepest gratitude to Sarah Ruth Gomes for graciously contributing her personal experience, strength and hope so vividly in the foreword to this book.

To Lois Bucco, RN, MS for her undying friendship, moral support and intuitive guidance for over twenty years.

To Kathy Bartow for her painstaking efforts as editor which consumed far more hours than were initially anticipated. While your intuition and suggestions improved this book immensely, your friendship is held in even higher regard.

My gratitude to Louisa Maisto, Darlene Smith, Ed Nyland, Thomas Weber at Cushing-Malloy, and Susie and Barb at Sans Serif for your encouragement, assistance and support.

My thanks to the following individuals for reviewing the manuscript prior to publication: Richard Bucco, MD, Josie Bucco, RN, Ed Epstein, DC, Karen Halpern, Esq., Patricia Hogan, RN, Marilyn Klainberg, EdD, RN, Stacey O'Connell, LCSW, Margaret Walker, RN, Lee Xippolitos, PhD, RN, Randy Scott Zelin, Esq., Art Zwerling, DNP, RN.

My list would be incomplete without crediting Divine Destiny with giving me a persistent vision of this book. Surely any capability or desire to write this never emanated solely from me.

Table of Contents

"If any feel that…we appear somewhat sentimental,

let them stand with us awhile on the firing line,

see the tragedies,

the despairing wives,

the little children;

let the solving of these problems

become a part of their daily work

and even of their sleeping moments…"

from Alcoholics Anonymous p.xxvi

Foreword

Becoming an expert in the tragedy of accidental overdose is nothing I asked for, or, before my mother's death, would have ever believed to be a possibility in my life. I had spent twenty-six years trusting in the strength of my mother, supported by her in countless ways, and admiring her accomplishments. You see, she was an amazing woman.

Her name was Jan Stewart. She was a nurse all my life. When I was four we moved from Washington to Rochester so she could study nurse anesthesia. After her graduation, we moved back to the Seattle area where she established her career as a Certified Registered Nurse Anesthetist (CRNA). She began work at a hospital where she would work for the next twenty years until her untimely death. Her commitment to the profession of nursing was extraordinary, culminating in strong advocacy and leadership roles within her hospital, as well as her state and national professional associations. Over the years she served on various committees and boards that promoted the profession and patient safety, including her leadership role as President of the American Association of Nurse Anesthetists (AANA) from 1999 to 2000.

Throughout her career, she never wavered in her commitment to raising me, giving me the space to grow into my own person, while staying close enough to be best friends. She also assumed leadership roles in organizations I was involved with while growing up. She was my chief seamstress for dance recital costumes, and my chauffeur to many rehearsals. She looked forward to my marriage and children with whom we planned her to have close involvement in raising.

It was during one of those many cross-country plane journeys during her service to the AANA, that she met a very special man. She had much to look forward to as they fell in love and planned a future together. Toward the end of her year as president she began to have intense back pain, but postponed needed surgery until she had completed her role. During that time she lived on airplanes, made numerous public appearances and endured lengthy meetings. Eventually she got back home, her surgery went well and she began setting up her new, more settled life in Seattle. She returned to a part-time position at the hospital where she'd worked for so many years and also maintained a private practice at a plastic surgery office where she was the sole anesthetist. She relished the increased clinical time with patients, which she still found to be the heart of her work.

It is hard to know exactly when the drug-use began, as no one knew about it until after her death. Perhaps it started with her back pain in 2000, or the pain medication she received for her surgery in 2001, or maybe it only started during her ultimate decline in the last few months of her life in 2002. However, careful reflection revealed the many warning signs of an impending problem, which led to the use. I saw many indications of my mom's illness but didn't know how to put them together until it was too late. I witnessed the signs of decline in her health…a gradual onset…layer upon layer. She would experience crippling headaches, nausea, out of character behavior, and eventually swollen hands and feet due to compromised veins. Near the end she suffered from deep bone pain, memory loss, and emotional imbalance.

The last time I spoke with her was a Wednesday evening, a short conversation as I was on my way to an appointment. She had another headache and said she was going home to take a shot and sleep. I never guessed that those shots were anything more than migraine medicine, but my inner-voice told me that tomorrow we must have further conversations about her health issues. But tomorrow never actualized for us. She died alone in her bed early the next morning of an accidental overdose of Sufentanyl. She had just turned fifty.

I'm not the only person who should have known more about what we observed. Even those who "knew better" didn't know enough to intervene in my mom's situation. The surgeon in her private practice was not surprised by her death because he had witnessed the telltale behavior, charting discrepancies, and other practice-related signs. We learned that others in their office, including administrative staff, saw signs of her illness and, like me, didn't know what to make of them. It is believed that mom had diverted the drugs that actually killed her from the hospital where she had worked that day. There she had known her colleagues for twenty years. Surely, they didn't know what to make of these signs, as she was a respected, long-time colleague and friend. Now of course, they too know that anyone can fall victim to the disease of addiction.

At times it's been easy to ask myself how none of us could have known. But what I've discovered is that these factors are not well known, especially to family. Even for other healthcare professionals, it is easy to believe that someone so effective and accomplished would never fall victim to such a disease. The SHUNT indicators outlined in this book have shed so much light on how someone like my mom was put in harm's way merely by participating in her profession. They succinctly summarize all of the indications leading to my mom's use that her family and friends have reflected upon over the years since her death.

One of my wishes is that no other nurse or their loved ones fall to this disease in the shadow of humility and misunderstanding. As this book highlights, the efforts to educate nurses about the possible danger of chemical dependency have fallen short of actually preventing use. The magnitude of the problem is significant. This book reminds me that with further preventative measures and widespread understanding, not only can we prevent death, but we may also be able to identify those at higher risk of using in the first place. This also gives me great hope for those who do find themselves in the chemical dependency trap, that there are ways we can support them to become healthy, productive individuals again.

I tell this story so that if you think you're immune to this disease and that you do not need to educate yourself on this subject, you will hopefully think twice. This book may save your life or the life of someone you care about. Little did I know that chemical dependency among nurses was so rampant. But, even if I did, I don't think I would have believed it could affect my mom. Like our family, in the blink of an eye, your life could be forever altered. I hope that you make yourself aware of the dangers and identify when there are increased risk factors so that you may help prevent the first use or know that intervention is necessary, should you be faced with someone in the grips of this disease.

Sarah Ruth Gomes

Preface

This book is based on what is commonly accepted as general knowledge of chemical dependency in the United States as a whole, and what I have observed specific to the nursing profession.

You may very well be asking yourself what qualifies me to write such a book. I asked myself the very same question as I embarked on this endeavor. In all honesty, it was my response to this query which ultimately propelled me forward, full steam ahead, on this project. Though somewhat typical of the nurse next door, my experience spans thirty-three years which have pivoted around chemical dependency.

My career began, like many other nurses, with a two-year stint in general medical and surgical nursing, as a staff nurse, in a New York City hospital. My assigned unit had the unenviable reputation as the last stop before heaven, due to the severity of our patients' conditions. Those outcomes, of course, were less than desirable.

Upon moving to a suburb about sixty miles away, I obtained a night shift position, working on a gynecological surgical unit. After nearly a year, I was enticed by supervisors to transfer to the

1

intensive care unit, where I had already been floating regularly.

Although not the focus of my career at this point, I encountered more than a fair share of chemically dependent patients, and worked with more than a few colleagues who had somewhat less obvious symptoms, but issues nonetheless.

I was hijacked, so to speak, in 1986 from the clutches of critical care, and began working in the psychiatric and detox units of the same hospital I had now been employed by for eight years. This transition was eagerly anticipated due to the effective lobbying efforts of a friend who worked in one of those areas. The availability of shorter shifts clinched my decision, as it better suited the needs of my young children.

A brief foray into occupational health in 1990, on a part-time basis, gave me a wider, more unique perspective on the impact of chemical dependency in the workplace. This, coupled with my interest in the field, prompted me to enroll in the South Oaks Institute for Alcohol and Addictive Studies in 1991, which proved to be an invaluable education.

Becoming nationally certified in addiction nursing the following year, I chose a brief sabbatical from the bedside. I commenced working as a public health nurse in the community, with an assigned territory which was notorious for drug abuse and related crimes. My primary duties revolved around making unannounced home visits to mothers whose newborns had tested positive for drugs and/or alcohol.

After conducting infant health assessments for nearly a year, an aunt offered to reimburse my tuition if I returned to school for an advanced degree. With that incentive, I reluctantly enrolled in graduate school in 1993. That the education was ultimately at my own expense proved to be just one example of destiny dangling a carrot in front of me, teasing me from hesitation into cooperation. As there was no specialty in addiction nursing, I chose the psychiatric and mental health track, by default.

During the two years of full-time course work, I continued working in the detox and psychiatric units of two hospitals on a per diem basis. In addition to classroom instruction, there were clinical rotations which prepared me for an advanced practice role. The final clinical practice segment was a full year's internship at a BOCES school. My function was to provide group and individual psychotherapy to emotionally disturbed female students. Not surprisingly, many of them had a component of substance abuse in the mix.

After graduate school, I set my sights on obtaining employment in an outpatient setting. This dream was realized in 1996 when I started working for a health information technology company. As a healthcare consultant, I provided strategic business decision support to various Fortune 500 clients regarding their human capital management programs. My interactions with various levels of management were centered on employee absence, illness and disability, as well as the risk of injury in the workplace. Much of these efforts were devoted to issues involving an employee's problem with chemical dependency, which had become evident in the workplace.

This experience provided a segue a year and a half later into a position as a Workers' Compensation field care manager for an insurance carrier's subsidiary. After a year, my career focus of chemical dependency began to share the spotlight with another specialty. This was not due to an innate interest on my part, so much as being identified by superiors as a good candidate for a company-sponsored training course in legal nurse consulting. This education signified me as one of a handful of nurses throughout the country who was able to provide a new product to defense attorneys and claims representatives.

Believing the theme of my career to now be more closely aligned with legal nurse consulting, I became nationally certified in that specialty in 2001. Were it not for a beautifully balmy day in autumn that year, I may well have remained in that position, indefinitely. But, as fate would have it, along with the Twin Towers went one of my employer's parent company offices. Much of their corporate fiscal strength crumbled along with those majestic buildings.

The aftermath of this tragedy catapulted me, at the request of my employer, into providing critical incident stress management services to those who had been on-site during the terrorist attack on September 11th. While all their employees had managed to physically escape the devastation, those individuals were by no means unscathed. For several weeks, I met daily with each displaced employee, in group and one-to-one sessions. My energies were devoted to maximizing their support systems, minimizing stress and recommending that all mood-altering substances be avoided, unless specifically prescribed by a physician.

At this time, I was also approached by an organization producing a public service television broadcast on stress reduction, in order to assist the public in coping after the incident. Invited as one of three expert panelists, one unanimous suggestion echoed by each of us was that the use of drugs and alcohol were not effective methods of dealing with the tension, anxiety and/or grief which many became intimately familiar with.

In December of 2002, I opted to resign from my legal nurse consulting role, as the dwindling referrals were unmistakably leading to layoffs. Six months later, I found myself on the doorsteps of a program exclusively devoted to chemically dependent nurses, whether or not the issue affected their profession. For more than five of the ensuing years, I focused solely on chemical dependency, as it pertained to nurses. I interviewed and worked closely with hundreds who were afflicted. I met with thousands of other individuals who had been impacted by the actions of the chemically dependent nurse on a personal or professional level, and provided education and referrals when necessary.

Along with assessing the chemically dependent nurses in-person, and providing periodic follow-up to those enrolled in the program, I met regularly with employers, treatment providers, attorneys and employee assistance program personnel on behalf of these nurses.

Upon request, I provided presentations on the risk of chemical dependency in the profession. The audiences were usually nurses whose employers had arranged for the session to be conducted at the workplace. Frequently, nursing instructors would incorporate the information into part of a class given to students at the nursing school.

Over the years, however, it became increasingly apparent that, in spite of giving these classes, which were geared towards the prevention of chemical dependency in the profession, some newly-trained nurses would require my services within a year or two post-graduation. It also became evident that some of their more seasoned counterparts would also fall prey to the chemical dependency trap, despite information given out on the subject. So, I began looking for similarities in the nurses who went on to encounter an issue.

After a time, I discovered the presence of several common denominators which were often obvious in nurses whose career had been encroached upon by substance use. A mental checklist of these characteristics began to form, based on the preponderance of these factors at the time of our initial meeting. Although the combination of traits varied, the vast majority of chemically dependent

7

nurses had at least two or more of these attributes displayed dominantly.

It was also noticeable that many of these same qualities became muted in recovering nurses, over time. Like clockwork, however, there was a corresponding rise in their prevalence prior to and during relapse.

While all of my education and professional experience qualify me to write this book, it offers the reader little, if any, explanation as to why I wrote this, or of who I am, at the core of my being.

Put simply, I have been the very closest of spectators to the anguish suffered by nurses caught in the cross-hairs of chemical dependency. I have found their pain unsurpassed by any other human condition. This speaks volumes when one considers my experience caring for those, critically ill and near death, for nearly a decade.

I can attest that the visible, audible and palpable devastation I have witnessed in five years working with chemically dependent nurses has totally and unequivocally eclipsed the cumulative tragedy I have observed in twice as many years working in ICU, medical, and surgical units.

The ripple effect on families, friends, co-workers, employers and society is of tsunami proportions. The damage to reputations is often irreparable. The fallout felt by households is frequently catastrophic. Although personally spared of all this, its proximity leaves me with a sense of personal responsibility.

I know, beyond any shadow of doubt, that the fate which befell any of these nurses could have been mine. Instead of the carrot of a fully funded master's degree dangled in my path, it very well may have been Vicodin, Oxycontin or Dilaudid that enraptured me.

When all is said and done, there are more similarities than differences among myself and every human being on the planet. My kinship with all nurses exists, regardless of any personal and professional distinctions. No matter what our age, ethnic background or native tongue, there is a common language of heart and spirit.

Thus, I know that the fate of any chemically dependent nurse could have been my own. Very easily, all too easily, in a heartbeat, I could have been another one added to the list. I also could have been one among the many, now dead, who lived far short of their natural life expectancy, directly or indirectly due to chemical dependency.

This book is not an appeal for sympathy, from any quarter; nor is it an attempt to levy blame on the nurses who have unwittingly become captives of the disease process of chemical dependency.

Several books and many articles have been written about chemically dependent professionals. Some have highlighted nurses, while others have placed little focus on them. With all due respect for the literary efforts of others, my goal is to fill a void that was not initially apparent to me in 2003. In fact, no hole was visible for the first two years I worked with these nurses.

I had naively thought that an hour's education on the risk of chemical dependency in nursing would be sufficient inoculation for nursing students. I had erroneously believed that a presentation highlighting the pitfalls within the profession would prevent the neophyte nurse from traversing the path that landed more seasoned comrades in trouble. Although this information may have spared some, many have succumbed to the lure, in spite of the advance notice.

Similarly flawed was my logic that the un-afflicted nurse, in practice for years or decades, would navigate safely about, once armed with sufficient knowledge about chemical dependency. Some may very well have done just that, with some future immunity, due to the material presented. Others would later profess recall of meeting me and hearing me speak, only to experience, in a very up-close-and-personal way, the troubling scenarios I had described.

Inaccurately, I also thought that facilities acquainted with the facts in this matter, would establish effective procedures for dealing with chemically dependent nurses. While many have done just that, to their credit, others have yet to institute best practices.

Each state has its own unique laws governing nursing practice. Approximately forty states have established programs which offer an alternative to discipline for some nurses who are affected by chemical dependency. These systems offer an alternative track, which may take the place of all or some of the professional charges the chemically dependent nurse may otherwise have faced. Depending on the situation, criminal proceedings may also be avoided to some extent.

The intent of such programs is to safeguard the public, rehabilitate the nurse and preserve a valuable resource, the nurse's career. In this way, chemically dependent nurses are leveraged into treatment, and monitored when they return to practice. Requirements are established by the alternative to discipline program, sometimes in conjunction with the nurse's chemical dependency treatment provider. Certain criteria must be met by the nurse, which are gradually lessened over a period of several years, depending upon the program's protocol.

Nursing education and experience have taught me skills in critical thinking; not the least of which is to question what I see and examine it further. This has led me to the conclusion that there is a definite need to be filled and a challenge to be met. There is a formidable obstacle to be overcome and it is not solely chemical dependency, per se.

A far greater hurdle than chemical dependency in the profession may very well be a lackadaisical approach. Half-hearted contentment, caused by a sense of futility at the magnitude of this problem, may dissuade keen eyes from taking a closer look at what currently exists. Thus resignation may ultimately be a more insurmountable stumbling block and problem than chemical dependency is.

Preface

Strides in the treatment of chemical dependency in nurses and safer return to work practices have undoubtedly been made over the years. In those accomplishments, however, we may have settled without sufficient objection for an ongoing high level of risk, to both the profession and the public.

I applaud the advances in early identification, optimal treatment and employer policies which support nurses in recovery, as well as the monitoring programs which structure a safer return to work for these individuals.

Any accolades, however, are silenced by the stark reality that many nurses are continuing to fall into the hidden trap of chemical dependency. This treacherous snare of potential risk for all nurses has yet to receive a spotlight flagging the danger sufficiently to steer more nurses away from harm.

If "Unbecoming A Nurse" ignites critical thinking, fosters positive change in policy, stirs anyone to support recovering nurses without moral judgment, and/or averts the disastrous spiral many have experienced, it will have served its intended purpose.

Introduction

Like most books, this one depicts a brief snapshot of time. The completion of this project required a sequence of actions almost too numerous to recall. One overwhelming sensation which was palpable throughout the entire process was an indelible feeling of urgency. Since this book's inception, there has been a rush of unrelenting energy beneath it, as well as behind it. This force created an unmistakably powerful momentum, like a strong wind, pushing me forward.

But, as I was re-writing the final version of these very paragraphs, I was struck with a need to pause, followed by an even greater commitment to seeing this project through to completion, as swiftly as possible.

My husband had just arrived home from work, with the first rendition of the book's front cover in his hands. Although he expressed praise regarding its appearance, he seemed a bit more somber than such an occasion called for. But no explanation was needed after he informed me that a woman at work had spied the cover, disclosing that her sister was a nurse living several states away. She then went on to reveal that this sister had recently lost a colleague from a suicide related to chemical dependency.

I do not believe that it is advancing age alone that makes the sting of such a tragedy so devastating to me. I cannot think of anyone who would not be equally alarmed upon hearing news of such an incident. Yet, this circumstance happens to an untold number of nurses and families, friends and employers, in every state. It is often overlooked, or misidentified, or swept under the rug, to protect reputations. Regardless of any of those particulars, all these situations are within a category I could only classify as heartbreaking.

Once, many years ago, I drove from my state of residence through the home state of the nurse that died so tragically. It was such a grueling ride that I swore I would never travel it by car, ever again. But it is not too far away to assuage the feeling of supreme sadness at the loss of this nurse. It strikes at my core, despite the distance, and hits me here, several states away, in the gut and the heart.

Although I have done my best to do this subject justice in an as-soon-as-possible time frame, this book will not reach the deceased nurse and loved ones quickly enough. But there are many more nurses and soon-to-be nurses, with their own collection of families and friends, who may benefit from this book. My sincerest hope is that others may bypass the hidden trap, which took the life of a nurse unknown to me, over a thousand miles away.

This issue is not unique to the borders of the United States. Chemical dependency abducts numerous nurses, as well as their children and closest contacts. It impacts friends, colleagues, employers and patients. A drain on our economy comes through lost productivity. If co-occurring physical and psychological ailments are taken into account, the price tag climbs even higher. The issue affects us all, although some feel the sting much more harshly, personally and permanently. Knowing no boundaries, taking lives in addition to hostages, and certainly offering no professional courtesies: that to me is a pretty apt description of chemical dependency.

Yet, many courtesies were afforded me upon embarking on this project. Sometimes they came unexpectedly from people I have never met. It seemed that at the crest of each challenge I encountered, there was a reciprocal fulfillment of whatever was needed, in the form of a gift, a solution or a message.

Introduction

Those around me may well have thought I'd lost
my senses; for in this economy, who would leave a
good-paying job and not pound the pavement for
another? It is in no small way the beneficence of
my husband which permitted me the latitude to
accomplish this endeavor. He willingly offered me
the seed money to self-publish this book, and the
funds to cover all household expenses during this
period.

There was the dear friend who graciously painted a
piece, specifically for the cover, which was
ultimately not used. The painting has a special
place in my office, a memento of the earliest days
of this project.

Another friend, skilled in editing, gave much of her
time, energy and effort to the project. The face,
hands and camera of another were borrowed for the
cover photo. Some professional contacts willingly
reviewed the manuscript, prior to printing and
graciously provided comments and suggestions.

Countless others freely donated moral and
technical support, in order to make this vision a
reality. There was the mother, with young children
underfoot, who patiently took me under her wing,
giving me a crash course on web pages, domain

addresses and other matters completely foreign to me.

At no time could I contemplate slowing down or turning back. Rather than sit on the sidelines and lament over the lives of those lost and wounded, I found myself unable to remain passively silent. There is a dire need that this subject be aired. This is in the best interests of all, myself included, in order that a collective intelligence, far greater than mine, may offer solutions not yet recognized.

This book imparts what is commonly known, as well as my professional experience, regarding chemical dependency in nurses. More questions may be raised than answered. The ultimate value of this book may be just that: to provoke thought.

Most studies have conservatively estimated that, within a nurse's lifetime, the incidence of a problem with drugs and/or alcohol will be ten percent or more. While similar rates occur in the general population, there are risks and consequences unique to nursing professionals.

Terms are plentiful describing alcoholism and drug addiction. Definitions abound in the often vain attempt to distinguish recreational use from dependence and abuse. This book is not meant to be a platform for debate regarding such matters.

Introduction

Throughout this book, the phrase "chemical dependency" has been chosen, because in my estimation it carries the least stigma. The term does not exclude any particular substance, be it licit, or illicit; socially accepted or objectionable. It includes all self-medication with mood-altering chemicals, regardless of whether they are prescribed, obtained over the counter, copped on the street, or procured via the internet. The use of antidepressants and other medications, which are taken as legitimately prescribed for their intended purpose, is not included in this definition.

Since the dawning of the 12-step movement of Alcoholics Anonymous, many individuals have viewed chemical dependency as a disease. I wholeheartedly concur with this belief. The chemical dependency process is certainly manifested by an inability to cease or moderate use of a substance, in spite of negative consequences. Often there is even a desire to stop, yet the pattern continues. The only logical rationale that adequately explains this repetitive cycle of behavior, which continues in spite of physical, emotional, financial and legal repercussions, is that a disease has taken hold. That these ramifications may end in loss of license, or even life itself, just adds weight to this opinion.

Most diseases are characterized by signs and symptoms. While some conditions have highly visible manifestations, others are known to fester in obscurity, out of sight. Sometimes, indications of chemical dependency may lurk in the shadows for years, prior to detection. Similar to other discreet disease processes, which are not prevented or treated in their infancy, the condition may progress, making it more difficult to obtain recovery.

While a protracted course of this disease is not uncommon among nurses, the nature of our profession can lead to an extremely rapid escalation of symptoms. Thus, nurses in a few weeks may reach levels of dependency which absolutely require an in-patient admission for detoxification. Often there is a fear of professional exposure if treatment were sought, and an incorrect belief that the nurse can manage their own withdrawal process. Like the physical law of inertia, in which an object's motion continues unless acted upon by a greater outside force, nurses often continue this downward trend, unless intervened upon by others.

In most diseases, there is an organ or system which is malfunctioning or negatively impacted by the condition. It could successfully be argued that in the case of chemical dependency, the brain is the region most affected. Therefore, it is not surprising to find that the thinking, judgment, insight and impulse control, which originate in the brain, are less than reliable in the chemically dependent nurse. Due to an inability to be objective regarding oneself, there is also little or no capacity to accurately assess one's situation.

Multiple factors predispose one to any ailment. Genetic, environmental and other variables play a role in increasing or mitigating the risk of becoming chemically dependent. The relationship of these components to elements found in a nurse's training, acculturation to the profession, and professional duties, is readily apparent. While no level of risk equates with an absolute certainty that one will succumb to any particular outcome, minimizing hazards is a large portion of what nurses do every day for patients. Yet, as nurses, we need to redirect some of this focus on prevention towards ourselves.

One of my utmost priorities throughout this book is to present chemical dependency in the nursing profession objectively and without moral judgment. Shame is not a prerequisite to victory over any obstacle or condition. Certainly, chemical dependency carries enough challenges without unnecessary stigma, which would further impede the recovery process.

The attitude proposed here is one of no blame. This position is not incompatible with holding a nurse accountable for behavior related to the chemical dependency. A well-planned intervention is the very best expression of living ethics, especially when it is done in a caring, decisive and nonjudgmental way. Without prompt intercession, many indeed may not live to reach their full potential or life expectancy. Therefore, taking a proactive stance, as quickly as possible after recognition of a problem, is a moral imperative.

The subject of this book may be unpleasant to many and unwelcome by some. In spite of that, there is an urgent need to highlight this topic, not only within the profession, but to the general public as well. Efforts have been extremely well-meaning to date, yet remain largely inadequate. In spite of the vigorous attempts of many, it seems so much more could be done.

I am at a blessed stage in life, which is due in no small measure to the gifts that this profession has given me. I invite you to take a close look at this topic, whether or not you have ever worn nursing shoes. Possibly, light will be shed on a subject, which may have been somewhat obscure. Hopefully, greater awareness will peak concern and interest, giving way to increased attention to this serious matter.

In a world where there are almost as many possible points of view as there are seats to view from, our combined talents, opinions and contacts can advance safeguards for all nurses and the public. I remain cautiously optimistic that, collectively, we may bring about whatever is necessary to prevent other tragedies, such as the one which recently provoked a nurse many miles away from me to commit suicide.

Becoming A Nurse

It is impossible to un-become any station or stage in life, prior to becoming. To arrive at the threshold of this profession, one must go through a myriad of steps in order to actually don the uniform and title of nurse.

My first experience with nurses was one of comfort, laced intermittently with dread. In the 1960's, I underwent an elective, non-emergency appendectomy. The surgery had been planned for weeks, and I was admitted to a hospital in Brooklyn, which no longer exists.

Forty-five years later, I still hold several extremely vivid memories, related to that one-week stay in a co-ed ward, with five other pediatric patients. There was the escapade with a wheelchair, commandeered by an older co-conspirator in the next bed, who wheeled me into an area strictly forbidden to us. The most delectable excitement from that wayward trip quickly turned to sheer terror when we were later discovered by an orderly. Due to past experiences with corporal punishment which was used liberally in those days, I feared we may both be carted back to the O.R. suite. This time it would be for surgery without parental consent, performed by an orderly who would disregard the Hippocratic oath, as he took a scalpel to our throats.

My most profound recollections, however, were three very stirring interactions I had with two nurses, who could only be described as polar opposites. The first, old and crotchety by any standards, was efficient, stern and technically proficient. Patient teaching, hand-holding and gentleness were not her strong suit. Her method of introduction came via a command, not a request, to roll on my side. Within moments of complying, my only awareness was a very uncomfortable sensation of being intruded upon, in areas never discussed at the dinner table. It was embarrassing beyond belief and totally unexpected. I became increasingly alarmed, as I feared I was about to undo the perfect record I had obtained regarding the proper use of toilet facilities. Needless to say, this was not a nurse I ever wanted to see again, let alone emulate.

Fortunately, this experience was followed by two extremely positive encounters with Kathleen. Though starched stiff as cardboard like her counterpart, Kathleen was young, pretty, and lit up the room with her smile. She was the epitome of wholesome. Here was a nurse who held my hand and soothed me through the dreadful ordeal of having abdominal sutures removed. It was Kathleen who bathed me tenderly my first day after surgery, taking time to apply the perfume I had been given by my grandmother the night before, as a get-well gift.

It was not until nearly a decade passed that I made, what was for me, the difficult decision to become a nurse. Believing that the best education was an absolute necessity, I explored the best four-year nursing programs offered at the time. There were two National League of Nursing accredited colleges nearby, both with excellent reputations, which I applied to.

Having chosen one to attend, some fellow classmates and I decided to vigorously petition for the ability to adjust our class schedule, in order to complete our baccalaureate degree in three years, plus a few months. By attending school four long, hot summers, and taking extra credit every semester, a handful of us obtained our degree in nursing, in August of 1975.

I have never regretted my decision to become a nurse, nor the choice to accelerate my educational experience. It did, however, take nearly twenty years for me to recuperate sufficiently from the experience before I could even contemplate obtaining an advanced degree.While completing nursing school and acquiring eligibility to sit for the state licensing exam are commendable accomplishments, they are a very far cry from actually passing one's nursing boards. Certainly, obtaining a nursing license is also quite praise-worthy, but this too is several light-years away from really becoming a nurse.

Becoming a nurse necessitates a thorough understanding of many scientific principles, including physics, anatomy, physiology, chemistry and pharmacology. It is about learning the dynamics of psychology and sociology. In decades past, as well as today, in spite of the advent of calculators, there is still a need to know at least the basic rudiments of mathematics.

But becoming a nurse goes far beyond this. Underneath all the principles is one that is irreplaceable, with no viable substitute: compassion. Becoming and being a nurse is all about being compassionate. Being a nurse is synonymous with caring. Becoming a nurse, therefore, has often been categorized as a calling. It requires commitment, character and integrity, which cannot possibly be gleaned from a book. Compassionate caring cannot really be taught, even by the most talented, dedicated and revered educators in the field.

Becoming and then being a nurse holds one to an extremely high standard of ethics; principles that are very difficult, at times, to adhere to. The expectations from employers, patients and our loved ones come perilously close to a perfection that is unattainable at times. Our expectations of ourselves often climb even higher than that.

It is the profession that has been said to "eat its young," while also being heralded as one that offers mentors and preceptors to help the less seasoned nurse.

What attracted me to the profession, beyond wanting to follow in Kathleen's footsteps of meticulous caring while soothing the wounds of others, was the diversity and dependability of work. Nursing is resilient. In the face of hard economic times, it offers a smorgasbord of experiences, at least one to satisfy any taste. The variety of work assignments, hours and locations is unsurpassed by any other profession. We work around the clock, all over the globe and in every industry, including the military. We have familiar practice areas, such as hospitals, nursing homes and clinics, as well as niche areas, such as consulting. We have been employed by film producers to ensure accurate portrayal of hospital scenes in the movies and television. We have become involved in public policy related to healthcare and have responded to natural disasters, as well as terrorist attacks.

Although dubbed "angels of mercy" by some, we are not saints. If we have any saintly quality, it is that, like saints, we keep on trying, in spite of our sins. While by and large compassionate and ethical, we are a profession at risk. It is common knowledge that nurses, increasingly, are the victims of workplace violence. As a group, we have greater exposure to virulent organisms and toxic substances than the general public. We are called upon to perform tirelessly and flawlessly, often with inadequate rest.

The list of possible rewards and potential hazards can be listed further, but is unnecessary for the purposes of this book. Suffice it to say that one does not become a nurse by chance or default. One becomes a nurse by a calling to make that decision; and once decided, one is required to set foot on a strenuous path of education, commitment and diligent practice.

Nowhere in this lengthy, very deliberate process does it ever dawn on any one of us to think or plan for a future "Unbecoming A Nurse."

Risk Factors

From conception, there is an element of possible risk associated with every activity. From infancy, we grow more accurate in our estimation of who, what, where and when we may encounter a potential threat to our well-being. At some point, we realize that even a state of inactivity offers no guarantee of safety, and often carries its own possible hazard.

In spite of modern advances and sophisticated technology, everyday life remains fraught with possible peril. We face potential injury while driving our cars, riding bicycles, rollerblading or taking in sites as tourists. Mishaps occur in our residences, whether they are our very own version of the American dream or the money pit. In a heartbeat, our lives can be forever changed by a missed step on a staircase or a ladder. Just as quickly, we can become injured using one of the many time-saving devices we use to beautify or maintain our home.

The use of chemicals to clean household surfaces may ultimately pose more danger to us than the bacterial colonies we try to banish from our bathrooms and kitchens. It also seems that our wide array of face, hair and beauty products may carry no less threat to our health and well-being when one examines the campaign for safer cosmetics underway in Europe. Obviously, carcinogens and noxious chemicals are much closer to most of us than previously imagined.

Certainly, ignorance does not truly equate to bliss in such a world where unsafe ingredients, which are in daily use, lurk inside our medicine cabinet, garage or kitchen cupboard. So, we follow closely the latest research on diet, exercise, health and safety warnings. We try to minimize our potential exposure by taking the best possible course of action and curtailing risky behavior. We conduct ourselves according to our own unique hierarchy of needs, desires and values, re-examining our lifestyle as we age and science advances.

Society, parents and big business have been in tacit agreement, cajoling and urging us to use caution while maintaining effective insurance coverage. In cases when we may have been less than prudent or just plain unlucky, we are courted to purchase various policies to protect anything and everything we cherish. Every few years, there is yet another offer for a product which can shelter us from yet another growing risk. Corporate underwriters establish new pricing guidelines, based on close analysis of the latest data on claims. Trends are tracked, and adjustments made accordingly, with an ever-growing litany of events and circumstances that may be excluded from coverage.

Meanwhile, loss prevention efforts continue to spawn the adoption of improved occupational safety protocols in every industry. Unfortunately, standards utilizing safer methods are often born out of tragic incidents which may still occur. Possibly unavoidable at the time, these events give rise to the adoption of even safer initiatives. Thus, the new procedures may take further aim at protecting employees, as well as the public and, ultimately, the corporate bottom line. The latest and most effective measures, however, are usually achieved at a price. The commitment of these expenditures from such limited resources as time, money and/or energy, is inevitable. In spite of this, the investment in best practices has come to be regarded by most as a necessity we would not want to do without. Rightly so, the personal and corporate value of "Safety First" often needs no justification.

Every line of work carries its own profile of risks versus benefits. Some roles engender the potential for chronic conditions, such as carpal tunnel syndrome in data entry personnel or knee problems in carpet installers. Some vocations are accompanied by conditions which decrease the quality, as well as length of life, such as steamfitters and ship builders exposed to asbestos. Even a heightened chance of sudden mortality, as well as morbidity, exists in some livelihoods, such as coal mining or construction.

Nursing certainly has its own intrinsic amalgam of advantages as well as drawbacks. Some are rather obvious, such as the possibility of an inadvertent needle stick while preparing or giving an injection. Virulent organisms, which are most resistant to the effects of antibiotics, are frequently less than an arm's length away for many nurses working at the bedside. Similar to other jobs, which require much lifting, nurses sustain a significant number of work related back injuries. Likewise, the vulnerability to workplace violence is higher in nursing than in many other professions.

Long known, yet less publicized, is the high rate of chemical dependency in nursing. Without close inspection of the variables within the profession which precede and/or increase susceptibility, there can be no evolution of optimal safeguards.

There is often, too, a propensity towards chemical dependency, which is evident in the background of some individuals, prior to high school graduation. The risk equation is comprised of many elements which are often independent of one's ultimate career choice. Therefore, any discovery analysis of the potential hazard, specific to any nurse, must begin with a brief look at some of the extraneous denominators which one may bring into the profession.

A strong family history has long been cited as a factor which increases the chance that one will succumb to many conditions. Certain types of cancer and heart disease are examples in which heredity plays a role. Chemical dependency is also known to have a genetic component, raising the likelihood of occurrence in those with close relatives who are, or were, afflicted. Of course, genes alone do not determine with absolute certainty whether any condition will occur. Distinguishing people who are at greatest risk, however, is significant because it enables more timely identification. When this translates into an earlier beginning of treatment, better outcomes are often attained.

In addition to heredity, certain personality traits seem to leave one more or less resistant to an alcohol or drug problem. Innate tendencies an individual may have towards impulsiveness, risk-taking and perfectionism are a few of the qualities which can be problematic. Without the benefit of an opposing trait to balance one's disposition, an individual may be drawn into precarious situations.

Environmental variables are also known to play a key role. These factors have greatest impact upon children and young adults. An absence of optimal nurturing in childhood is often accompanied by an inability to adequately self-soothe later in life. This may lead some to seek consolation in mood-altering substances. Those raised without the benefit of effective role models during their formative years may lack the coping skills required to tolerate the frustrations of everyday life. The onslaught of peer pressure, which frequently precipitates a young person's initial alcohol or drug use, may prove irresistible in such cases.

Growing up in homes riddled with alcohol or drug problems often slants one's perception of what constitutes "normal" behavior. Many do become aware that they possess a skewed view of life. As a result, they aptly describe their family of origin by the cliché "dysfunctional family." Few would disagree that the person emerging from this environment embarks on life at a certain disadvantage. Such a handicap goes far beyond any personal choice to refrain regarding alcohol and drug use. While some may swear off entirely, others go on to closely model the behavior they witnessed in parents or guardians.

Many adult children of alcoholics and drug addicts exit such households with the belief that they have escaped these environments unscathed. In spite of a change in zip code many find, especially around midlife, that their biological family drives their decision-making and lifestyle choices. This is often true, regardless of whether any may have acquired their own problem with chemical dependency.

Another indicator of risk is early and extensive substance use. The brains of young people are much more susceptible to the effects of drugs and alcohol than adults. Chemicals used while the brain is still maturing can alter the developing brain. These changes are considered by many experts to be irreversible. Thus, the earlier in life one begins alcohol or drug use, and the more extensive such use becomes, the greater the impact on the brain.

Added to any underlying circumstances which predispose an individual towards chemical dependency are several components of risk inherent in the nursing profession. Many have gravitated to this profession because its hallmark prerequisites are compassion and sensitivity to the needs of others. Regardless of whether these traits are already overdeveloped in a person prior to entry into the profession, we strive to exemplify and amplify these qualities to the highest degree possible.

We then marry this acute sensitivity and ability to hone into the plight of others, with the inescapable necessity of being closely intertwined with patients for extended periods of time. Thus most full-time nursing roles demand roughly forty hours per week immersion in a bath of pain, suffering, sorrow, tragedy and sometimes death. The product of our training, combined with this exposure, melds into an often unacknowledged acquisition of second-hand trauma.

Like those serving in combat, we are taught to keep very tight reins on our feelings. In disciplined fashion, we contain any verbal or bodily clue which would mirror the patients' suffering back to them. We keep a lid on telegraphing signals of any troublesome complications which would be alarming to patients or their loved ones. We keep our calm exterior and smile intact, in spite of sights, smells or sounds, which in any other circumstance would require quite a different response.

Inherent in military and police efforts is an education and training goal of officer safety, while in our role there is less attention to self-care. Where soldiers and law enforcement officers have the release valve of aggression in the face of danger or distress, nurses are afforded no such safety mechanism. It is at these times that we often make the misguided assessment that "we can handle it," denying to our innermost selves a need for ongoing support. While debriefings are an essential strategy for our brothers and sisters in the military, they are often lacking on the firing line of the nursing profession. Intellectualizing, we unwittingly override any human being's capacity for empathy. Thus, we unknowingly add to our growing compost of what has recently been termed "compassion fatigue."

This list of pertinent risks would be incomplete without a close look at the education which enables us to meticulously care for patients. Much of our schooling pivots around one of the most routine and important tasks nurses perform daily in most practice areas: the safe and effective administration of medication. This learning provides us with detailed information about potent chemicals, many of which are habit-forming. We gain mastery in handling, preparing and giving these potions, as well as making astute observations of the effects they have on the recipient. Increasing adeptness at these skills, over time, naturally lends itself to a normal routine of familiarity and de-sensitization. The once very deliberate and somewhat stressful task of medicating patients has now, by sheer repetition, become natural, methodical and largely predictable. This subtle comfort regarding our knowledge and clinical expertise leads to a certain sense of invulnerability.

During our initial schooling as nurses, little attention may have been given to the enhanced risk of chemical dependency within our profession. Moreover, any education we did receive in this area may have been replaced by the scar tissue of self-regard for our expertise with medication administration. We continually monitor our medicated patients closely, taking appropriate measures based on our findings. We accurately communicate information as needed, acting as liaisons between doctors and patients. For the most part, it is our feedback, based on a combination of direct observations of our patients and the instincts we develop with clinical experience, which assists the prescribing physicians in making accurate medication adjustments.

The hidden trap, which any nurse can fall prey to, is that our education and experience in safely and effectively medicating patients somehow qualifies us to safely and effectively self-administer these same substances. These thoughts may sometimes meet with little or no resistance. We may well have been lulled by our own proficiency in medicating our patients. The illusion that one's knowledge about addictive substances serves as a barrier or vaccine against becoming addicted actually serves to increase, rather than decrease our risk.

What escapes the self-medicating nurse's awareness is the fallacy in this thinking. This flawed thought process often goes undetected by the nurse. Clear insight and sound judgment is lost as to the repercussions of such actions. At the very moment self-medication takes place, there is the total annihilation of any bona fide caregiver who is in attendance. This lack of qualified professional observer is of great concern. With no one on-call to monitor and protect the nurse, who has now become the pseudo-patient, a serious threat exists, which may go undetected for some time.

The potential for jeopardy may also exist related to merely handling and administering medication. In the past, we have thought we knew much in some subjects, only to later discover misconceptions in our understanding. For example, the belief that hormone replacement therapy lowered multiple risk factors in menopausal women was amended, based on additional research. Therefore, an absolutely risk-free method of delivering potent chemicals may later be deemed inadequate in fully protecting nurses.

Possible hazards accompanying the duties of medication administration may deserve a cautionary note, in spite of any assurances from manufacturers. Not long ago, we may have believed that providing anesthesia at the head of the operating table could not possibly inadvertently deliver the sedative, by way of second-hand exposure, to the anesthetist. Far from science fiction, however, this can happen. The ultimate unpredictability of inadvertent exposure was overlooked by Chechen rebels who anesthetized a whole theater full of people in Russia several years ago. The unintended death of many during that incident has prompted questions by many regarding any assumptions we might make about safety in handling substances and the possibility of unknown exposure and risk to nurses.

In spite of the previously mentioned occupational threats, if one feels called to the nursing profession, one does not usually explore an alternate career path solely because of an elevated potential for harm. Whether the possibility of danger comes from an inadvertent needle puncture, back injury or other job-related exposure, including chemical dependency, one tends to utilize utmost precautions and reap great fulfillment from the profession of nursing.

Just as fair-skinned individuals' exposure to sunlight poses a potential threat of skin cancer, many nurses may remain vulnerable to chemical dependency to some degree. While the fairest will continue to venture into the sunlight, so too will at-risk individuals continue to enter the nursing profession.

The crusade against skin and other cancers has accomplished much in the way of informing the public. Pushing the limits of current knowledge, additional research is giving way to changes in behavior and more accurate methods of detecting the disease. Somewhat similar to cancer in its invasiveness and destructiveness is the disease of chemical dependency. Like cancer, it can impact more people than those who fall victim to it. Certainly the lives of those diagnosed with either condition are altered, sometimes with an improved ability to prioritize and appreciate life. Both conditions can also impact family members, often markedly and forever. Neither disease leaves friends, co-workers or employers unaffected. Whether a treatment provider specializes in cancer or addiction, there is great satisfaction in the tales of success, as well as great sadness for those lost in spite of efforts aimed at recovery.

Because of the incidence of chemical dependency in the profession, an acute need for proactive measures is warranted. Education which falls short of enlightening one sufficiently to amend attitudes and behaviors does not do justice to the profession, the nurse or society. Particularly if information leads one to an appraisal of innate invulnerability, rather than a greater appreciation of inherent weakness, the fund of knowledge can prove to be woefully incomplete, as well as potentially lethal.

The need for early and ongoing self-survey by nurses, aimed at the earliest possible discovery of any tendency towards traits frequently found in the chemically dependent nurse seems evident. The identification of those who are at greatest risk of succumbing to the disease, prior to an untoward event in the workplace, is critically important. This may allow some to bypass the chemical dependency trap altogether, or at least in part. In light of the danger to some who will eventually progress to have a serious issue, however, the custom of self-survey should be made as familiar to nurses as using a stethoscope.

The following chapter will focus on use of a screening tool I developed, which may help nurses measure their own risk of becoming chemically dependent. This self-appraisal is based on ten characteristics I frequently observed in chemically dependent nurses over the past five years. These attributes are present to various degrees in nurses not affected by chemical dependency and who may never have a problem in their lifetime. However, every single nurse who ever required my advocacy in a professional capacity related to chemical dependency possessed a very clear abundance of these traits at the time of our initial interview.

Risk Assessment

Informal screening tools have been in use for many years. They have been created to detect the presence of indicators which often accompany many conditions, including depression, anxiety and alcohol abuse. They have been used increasingly because they have provided earlier identification of those most likely to encounter an issue. The use of these instruments has improved outcomes in many situations and has prevented many worst-case scenarios.

The value of these instruments is undeniable when it steers those at greatest risk towards treatment sooner, rather than later. One such example is checking depressed individuals for the likelihood that they will attempt suicide. In many cases, this has indicated those at greatest risk of harming themselves, permitting prompt intervention, which has averted many from taking their lives. The result is that many have been prevented from taking their lives. The presence of heightened risk never predicts with absolute certainty that harm will occur. Nonetheless, we have accepted this uncertainty and continued to use screening tools, in the interest of safety.

Prevention and early intervention strategies have become the standard in healthcare. The ideal situation is when high blood pressure is treated before the occurrence of a stroke. Because high cholesterol levels have been correlated to the risk of heart attack, it has become customary to prescribe medication lowering the amount of cholesterol in the blood. This more aggressive management is recommended, even though there are many possible side effects, due to the large number of lives which may otherwise be lost to heart disease.

Annual PAP smears are urged in all women, because they can detect cervical cancer in the earliest, most treatable stage. Most people are strongly encouraged to have a colonoscopy by age fifty or prior to that time if there is a family history. All who have undergone PAP and colonoscopy exams will attest to the invasiveness of these procedures. In spite of that, they are performed regularly, because they may save the lives of many who would progress to an untreatable stage of cervical or colon cancer prior to detection. In many instances, insurance companies cover these tests, as cost benefit analysis confirms that the screenings save money, as well as lives.

Nurses are not exempt from any situation or illness. Our vocation gives us no professional courtesy. We are certainly not immune from becoming chemically dependent. As discussed earlier, our professional scope actually offers us avenues into chemical dependency which the general population does not gain access to. As indications of an issue often surface in the home or social arena before they become apparent at work, it is of vital importance to move up the timeline of identification. Thus, measures can be taken to effectively prevent incidents in the workplace.

While focusing on those who have already displayed a problem with chemical dependency is important, this is a retrospective tactic. To effect the greatest improvement in the situation, we must begin to implement methods which preempt the development of the condition, prior to the advent of a troubling incident. Such proactive measures should be aimed at all nurses and student nurses.

Though it remains crucial to deal with and adequately support nurses who already have a chemical dependency, we also need to give due diligence to tackling the high overall occupational exposure. The potential implications to the nursing profession, individual nurses, employers and society demand no less than utilization of any method which recognizes those at greatest risk, long before there is any hint of difficulty in the workplace.

It is with these facts in mind that I suggest the use of the screening tool presented here. The SHUNT Self-Survey For Nurses evolved as a natural outgrowth of the repeated similarities I observed over a five-year period, working exclusively with chemically dependent nurses. As time passed, a preponderance of these characteristics became strikingly familiar, regardless of the substance used. The nurse's age, gender and number of years in practice were seemingly irrelevant. Indicators were apparent in nurses who had an issue of only a few weeks' duration, as well as those who identified a long-standing problem of several years. The characteristics were present to a greater extent in those still self-medicating.

Many of these same attributes found on initial assessment decreased over time, as optimal treatment was engaged in and recovery milestones met. The traits continued to be less pronounced in nurses who fully integrated formal treatment recommendations into their lives. In nearly every case, the directives from chemical dependency treatment providers included regular participation in the 12-step programs of Alcoholics Anonymous and/or Narcotics Anonymous.

Conversely, the traits which had faded with treatment, 12-step involvement and abstinence from substance use, tended to become more apparent, prior to the occurrence of a relapse. Sheer elimination of substance use after a relapse did not necessarily equate to a complimentary decrease in these characteristics. However, when nurses stopped substance use, re-engaged in formal treatment and 12-step support, and complied with the recommendations given by those resources, the overall presence of traits receded once again.

This tool does not meet the strict criteria of scientific study, as validation and statistical significance have not yet been measured. Future research may be conducted which improves upon this survey. In the interim, however, self-survey by all nurses and nursing students seems advisable. Without an alternative device specifically designed to detect the risk of chemical dependency in nurses, before any problem is evident, this method should be utilized.

Those discovering the presence of many indicators on self-appraisal may be spared the personal and professional anguish which many chemically dependent nurses have experienced. Hopefully, such recognition will be made prior to the occurrence of a workplace incident. This is only the barest beginning at a preemptive approach which seems long overdue.

The self-assessment can be done quickly and easily by any nurse in less than five minutes. It may also be discussed with those closest to a nurse, such as a significant family member or friend. The greatest benefit may be achieved by those who have identified an issue with chemical dependency if this survey is completed in the company of their significant other, treatment provider or 12-step sponsor. This may eliminate the tendency of nearsightedness one seems to have regarding one's own risk. Looking at these traits together with a supportive individual may lessen any denial which may be present. Too many chemically dependent nurses already highlight the fact that those affected are often the last to see any elevation of risk or deterioration in behavior.

Ongoing self-survey of all nurses is recommended, regardless of whether a previous problem with alcohol or drugs has been recognized. For those with a past issue, however, the tool may highlight behaviors and circumstances which may lead one towards a relapse. While some nurses' stories of sobriety do include relapse, relapse is never a requirement for ongoing recovery. The path to relapse, although varied, has been very well charted and documented. While some may experience it, avoidance at all costs is a much better alternative.

The benefit to students from an early self-appraisal, preferably prior to enrollment in nursing school, is enormous. Along with ongoing educative efforts, the practice of regular self-survey may foster the development of protective behaviors which prevent negative consequences. Inclusion of family, spouse and/or friends in this process is encouraged as it provides the highest level of safeguards going forward.

The SHUNT Self-Survey For Nurses has a total of ten components. These items are not listed in any particular order of priority. Each letter stands for two separate characteristics, which may or may not be present in a nurse's current life. Only two of the traits have an element of permanence, as they pertain to historical events. This means that these two attributes, once scored affirmatively, will always require a positive response.

The tool is a very simple guide for identifying the presence or absence of indicators which are often found in chemically dependent nurses. Over time, the profile of any nurse may change, as lifestyle is altered or circumstances develop. This appraisal is not a diagnostic test, nor is there a score which indicates absolute risk. What the tool does offer, however, is a method by which one may recognize a preponderance of factors which may be leading one towards a problem with chemical dependency. This allows one the opportunity to make timely behavioral changes which minimize that risk.

The SHUNT Survey For Nurses is as follows:

S - Social withdrawal or self-isolative behavior.

S - Self-care behaviors beneath societal, professional or the nurse's own standards.

H - History of chemical dependency in the nurse's immediate family.

H - History of negative consequences related to the nurse's substance use.

U - Untreated or unremitting emotional or physical pain.

U - Using medication for a reason it was not intended or in a manner not recommended.

N - Nursing practice routinely in excess of fifty-five hours per week.

N - Nursing duties include frequent access to controlled substances.

T - Transitional period requiring major adjustment within the past year.

T - Turmoil or tragedy with unresolved conflict.

Scoring the survey is a simple matter of addition. The absence of any trait would be rated as a zero, while its presence would be scored as a one. The total possible score will range anywhere from zero to ten on the survey. Lower totals indicate less presence of risk factors, while higher values indicate a greater presence of risk factors. No score indicates a total absence of risk, or a certainty that one is, or ever will become, chemically dependent. The tool is not intended to diagnose chemical dependency or any other situation or condition. For convenience, a SHUNT Self-Survey For Nurses Scoring Sheet is located at the back of this book.

The first "S" trait, social withdrawal or self-isolative behavior, may elicit an affirmative response if the nurse has been an integral part of a group and is now on the periphery. Declining a large portion of invitations which would customarily be accepted by a nurse over a prolonged period, may rate a one. Examples may include participation in family, social or athletic functions. A nurse who has opted out of clubs, religious services or other organization, which were previously attended regularly, without adequate explanation, would fit this category. If the activities provided support or a pleasurable outlet, or served a purpose of high priority to the nurse, a score of one may be appropriate.

If association with others is minimized in order to hide symptoms of chemical dependency, this trait would merit a point. A compelling sign which demonstrates this attribute would be secretive behavior, including lies of omission as well as commission. As substance use becomes more habitual and pronounced, the nurse may make attempts to camouflage, minimize or hide any evidence of an issue. This is especially true regarding those closest to the nurse, such as friends and family members.

While no one escapes our modern world without occasionally being less than candid, one of the hallmarks of increasing dependence on substances is the tendency towards deception. Thus, hiding substance-related behaviors, and preventing loved ones from witnessing them, is a very telling sign. Therefore, if actions signify propulsion towards isolation and seclusion with a corresponding withdrawal from friends and relative, the first "S" factor deserves a rating of one.

The second "S" characteristic, self-care beneath societal, professional or the nurse's own standards, may be evident in a nurse who customarily practices good hygiene and lets appearances slide for an extended length of time. The nurse who goes without getting a front cap replaced or is in obvious need of other dental care for months, with no rationale for skipping treatment, may deserve a point. Similarly, the nurse who has time and money to lavish on others, yet telegraphs an ignorance or indifference to his or her own need for food, sleep, rest and recreation for long periods is another example.

Nurses who are accustomed to keeping their homes, cars or other possessions in good condition may begin to lack the awareness, energy or motivation to consistently sustain these efforts. When chemical dependency becomes apparent, it is not unusual for what one once valued to be relegated to the back seat.

Important responsibilities which cannot be

delegated to another or which one must personally initiate, such as legal or financial matters, may be ignored. A nurse who becomes unreliable or less punctual regarding the filing of tax returns, resolving traffic tickets or fulfilling other compelling obligations may be included here, if alcohol or drug use appears to be the cause.

The first "H" factor, a history of chemical dependency in the nurse's immediate family, is fairly straightforward. A point should be scored for this section if the nurse's biological parents, grandparents or siblings have had a problem with drugs or alcohol at any time during their life. If an issue ever existed in any close biological kin who are deceased or in recovery this section would still be scored affirmatively.

If a nurse discovers the existence of chemical dependency in the immediate family after the initial SHUNT survey, future assessments should be adjusted to reflect a positive response. Once present, this trait persists, in spite of any alteration in the family dynamics. As the only SHUNT indicator based on heredity, it is irreversible.

The second "H" trait, history of negative consequences related to the nurse's substance use, would include any criminal activity related to chemical dependency, regardless of the outcome. Driving while under the influence or intoxicated, possessing a controlled substance or forging a prescription while under the influence would score a point. Commission of any crime in order to obtain a substance, or due to impaired judgment, would also warrant a point. Domestic or other violence, child endangerment or neglect, disorderly conduct and/or harassment are some examples of situations which may be related to the actual use of substances and would warrant a point.

Performing acts of prostitution or theft, as well as selling drugs in order to have the necessary funds to procure one's own supply of substances would be rated affirmatively. Any charge which was reduced to a lesser offense or dismissed due to attorney representation, plea bargaining or a technicality, would also apply under this heading, regardless of any court ruling.

Not all negative consequences related to chemical dependency proceed to criminal or family court. Undesirable repercussions may reverberate in the nurse's professional life. Even if a nurse's actions occur outside the work setting, nurses are often held to a moral character clause. Normally, actions taken by a layperson outside of work would not impact their career. However, as nursing licensure is a privilege which holds one to additional standards, any actions taken by a nurse at any time may spark an investigation by the state licensing agency.

Charges levied against a nurse's license related to the habitual use of substances would therefore be included in this category. Any conduct which opposes the code of ethics of the American Nurses Association and/or the applicable state nurses' association would also qualify. Any termination, demotion or suspension by an employer which is related to the use of substances would also meet the criteria for this section.

The loss of one or more significant relationships due to chemical dependency would be another example of negative ramifications, even though no professional, civil or criminal charges may be involved. Loss of a loved one's trust, respect or continued affiliation certainly qualifies as an undesirable consequence. Any behavior which compromises one's values and moral beliefs may also be noted as an affirmative response under this heading.

Material losses, such as damaged automobiles or being placed in an assigned risk category for insurance coverage, would rate a point. Loss of physical health, including falls or other injuries, seizures, liver problems or complications from existing conditions due to chemical dependency would be applicable under this heading. Finally, exposure to a sexually transmitted disease or to an unwanted pregnancy due to risky behavior while under the influence would also merit a point.

The first "U" characteristic, untreated or unremitting emotional or physical pain, is often present in chemically dependent individuals, regardless of their occupation. Almost everyone will, over the course of a lifetime, sustain injuries or acquire conditions which cause pain. While symptoms may not immobilize us, they may very well alter our level of functioning and/or our ability to cope with other stressors.

Pain which goes unabated for a significant length of time, regardless of the cause, often prompts one to seek relief. This is extremely pertinent for nurses, who are often only an arm's length away from remedies which work wonders for patients. Therefore, pain or significant discomfort which is present for an extended period of time, without resolution, is a highly significant finding.

Since nursing is such a physically demanding

occupation, nurses may acquire work-related musculoskeletal injuries. Sometimes the cause may be strenuous physical exercise or another form of overexertion. Sometimes this is complicated by inadequate physical conditioning or advancing age. Motor vehicle as well as other accidents may also precipitate trauma which does not resolve quickly. Some common areas prone to injury are the back, neck, shoulders, knees, wrists and ankles. Nurses who have persistent symptoms related to trauma which persist without relief would score a point for this section.

The litany of physical conditions provoking pain without any traumatic event is quite long. Some noteworthy ones are migraine headaches, fibromyalgia and rheumatoid arthritis. While nurses may receive adequate relief, there should be vigilance in these situations because exacerbation of symptoms may occur. Therefore, if pain becomes difficult to manage, this category would require an affirmative response.

Not all unremitting or untreated pain, however, is physical in nature. Those with depression, anxiety or manic depression can attest to how extreme emotional symptoms can become. Often they rival any physical complaints nurses may experience.

Yet, sometimes the nurse may be unaware of the intensity of emotional distress, deferring formal evaluation and expert care. If any of these happen to be the case, the first "U" trait would score a point.

All emotional symptoms are not necessarily related to any innate chemical imbalance. Nurses who have become the victims of physical and/or emotional abuse may find their physical trauma was a simpler matter to heal. Situations related to natural or man-made disasters, such as earthquakes or the terrorist attack on the Twin Towers, may have longstanding implications for some nurses on an emotional level. All these as well as similar circumstances would fulfill the requirements of this section.

Another situation which applies to this section is prolonged difficulty sleeping. While the condition is not new to humanity, it has been long overlooked. Yet, it poses a real threat to health and safety for those with pronounced and prolonged sleep disorders. Therefore, if the condition persists unrelieved, a score of one is warranted.

There are many more conditions which are accompanied by any number of excruciating or annoying symptoms. Whether the diagnosis has been determined, if a condition remains or becomes troublesome for a prolonged period, without respite, this category would require a point.

The second "U" trait in the survey is using medication for a reason it was not intended for or in a manner not recommended. Nurses who continue using pain medication after symptoms have subsided would score a point. This would include increasing the dosage amount or frequency beyond the manufacturer's or physician's instructions. Using several medications which should not be combined would require an affirmative response. Likewise, using alcohol or other substances which may potentiate or compete with any prescribed or over-the-counter medication would indicate the presence of this trait.

This category differs from the first "U" trait because that reflects the objective presence of an underlying pain, psychological or other syndrome. The inherent risk in the former "U" category is that one may be provoked to self-medicate actual pain, discomfort and/or emotional distress, either intentionally or subconsciously. While the nurse may or may not be aware of the severity of symptoms, there is astute recognition of the powerful potions within reach. Treatment may be entirely absent if the nurse's symptoms have not led to formal evaluation. At other times, care may have been initiated, but relief of symptoms may be insufficient.

By comparison, the second "U" trait is the nurse actually self-medicating or manipulating the effect of medication with other chemicals. It may be one or a combination of substances which are taken in a manner unintended by the manufacturer or prescriber. Sometimes the precautions given by treating physicians or on the warning labels provided by drug companies and pharmacists are disregarded. Continuation of medication beyond the time it is needed, or adding alcohol or another substance to potentiate or alter the intended effect, would be included here.

The following examples will serve to illustrate the difference between both U traits. The first nurse medicates post-operative knee pain long after cessation of symptoms and in the absence of any other underlying physical or emotional conditions. This nurse would rate a score of one for the latter U category, but a zero for the former U trait.

A second nurse with post-operative knee pain has been treated with antidepressants for five years. This nurse stopped antidepressant medication a year ago, in spite of ongoing symptoms of depression. When knee pain ceased the third day after surgery, all medication was discontinued. This nurse would merit a zero for the second "U" characteristic and a one for the former "U" trait.

A third nurse who underwent knee surgery has no chronic underlying syndrome present and ceased all pain medication the second day after surgery when symptoms subsided. A score of zero for both "U" factors would be warranted.

A fourth nurse has self-medicated anxiety symptoms with alcohol for the past ten years without ever having a formal evaluation for this problem. Pain medication has continued for several months in spite of no lingering knee symptoms since the first week after surgery. This nurse would receive a point for both "U" categories.

The first "N" characteristic, nursing practice routinely in excess of fifty-five hours per week, is fairly straightforward. Consistently working more than fifty-five hours per week in a nursing role would rate a point for this section. Most full-time nursing positions usually equate to roughly thirty-five to forty hours weekly. To consistently work more than fifty-five hours per week equates at the very least to a thirty percent increase over full-time status requirements.

A nurse who works twelve-and-a-half-hour shifts may be scheduled to work fifty hours one week, and twenty-five hours the next week, to reach the hours needed for full-time employment in a particular position. This is not problematic because the period of fifty hours is balanced by a lighter schedule the subsequent week. Even in cases where the nurse may elect to work two additional twelve-and-a-half-hour shifts over a two-week span, the average hours worked would consistently remain beneath the fifty-five hours per week mark.

Regardless of the role any nurse fulfills, professional demands are steep and frequently accompanied by stress. "Burnout" is a term often used by nurses in every specialty to describe the overwhelming exhaustion experienced in the workplace. It is one of the top reasons given by nurses for exiting the profession prior to the customary retirement age.

The risk which accompanies excessive work is that a substantial increase in professional duties tends to detract from a nurse's ability to obtain adequate rest and recreation. Healthy pursuits which promote optimal well-being and fortitude may be curtailed or suspended entirely in favor of excessive work. Routinely working more than fifty-five hours usually requires a complimentary shift in other activities, which often equates to a significant decrease in recuperative time. This tends to add a burden of risk, thereby warranting a point.

The second "N" component, nursing duties include frequent access to controlled substances, identifies those in closest proximity to substances known to be habit-forming. Like all the previous variables noted, this one does not indicate that a problem is certain to occur. All studies point to the fact that the vast majority of nurses do not encounter a problem with chemical dependency. Yet, the hazard inherent in the nursing profession is greater than in many other occupations, particularly regarding controlled substances. It is commonly accepted that a greater element of this risk exists in nursing positions where there is the most frequent administration of these chemicals.

In assessing whether this factor rates a point, a nurse should evaluate whether there is a preponderance of pain management or sedation of patients in their job duties. Consideration should also be given to whether the standards at the workplace are sufficient to provide adequate protection to the nurse. Lax oversight of controlled substance waste procedures would be one example which may prompt a nurse to rate this category affirmatively.

Inadequate supervision or practice in isolated settings may also pose a hazard, especially if the patients cared for are unable to speak or advocate for themselves. A nurse responsible for destroying expired medications or who must draw medications from multi-dose vials on a consistent basis may also merit a point.

Nurses who become aware that they may have selected a setting or scope of practice consciously or inadvertently that affords greater access to controlled substances would be wise to score this section affirmatively. If there is a lack of scrutiny by others, caution may be indicated at the very least. In solitary contemplation, if a nurse finds the choice of assignment is related to having increased access to controlled substances or less oversight, wisdom would dictate identifying a practice setting with less exposure.

The first "T" factor, transitional period requiring major adjustment within the past year, would include a pending or recent marriage, separation or divorce or relocation of residence. Other changes would include having new job duties or a new employer, the birth of a child or death of a loved one. Graduate nurses and those who may have progressed to a more advanced practice role, as well as those about to retire, would also rate a point.

While many changes are positive and looked forward to eagerly, the requisite adjustment in lifestyle is nonetheless stressful. Therefore, regardless of how the nurse perceives the situation, if the change demands any significant alteration in routine or responsibilities, the category would be scored affirmatively.

The second "T" category, turmoil or tragedy with unresolved conflict, would encompass ongoing marital problems or difficulties with children or parents. The presence of a chronic or progressive illness in a loved one or dependent, such as dementia, ADHD or a stroke, would be included here.

Extreme financial hardship, being the victim of a crime or a witness to violence may prompt one to add a point to the survey. A nurse's behavior or that of someone close to the nurse which results in mass media attention, such as a scandal, may be included in this category. Especially if there is an impact on a nurse's reputation, this trait is evident. Loss or imminent curtailment of a license to practice nursing, whether surrender is voluntary or mandatory, would be marked affirmatively in this section.

Major unresolved conflict for some nurses surrounds an attempt to effectively balance professional and parental or other obligations. Any situation which leaves one with little hope of a viable solution, stresses one to the brink of hopelessness or causes ongoing guilt or shame, would meet this category's criteria, thus adding a point for this section.

Upon completing this self-survey with a response of zero for the absence of any trait and one point for the corresponding presence of any trait, all ten scores should be added. As mentioned earlier, the total will range from zero to ten. The lower the total, the fewer indicators of risk present. Higher numbers equate to a greater presence of risk factors.

Given that change is the only constant in life, a score of two this year may be quite different six months or a year from now. Ongoing risk appraisal would be helpful in identifying those with the highest ratings. Also of import are those with a significant elevation in risk factors over a period of time. This is crucial, because only two of the characteristics assessed are impossible of receding once they become apparent. Heredity cannot be changed, nor can one undo a history of a negative consequence related to chemical dependency. Yet, while these two factors, once present, will necessitate no less than a score of two going forward, all other characteristics can be moderated by behavior or the use of increased coping skills which enhance well-being.

The following chapter identifies optimal safeguards which may be helpful in decreasing any potential hazard of chemical dependency a nurse may face. Any practices which shield a nurse from developing an issue, serves to protect the public as well. Therefore, enacting any measures which support such endeavors would be well worth any necessary commitment of time, energy and/or money.

Optimal Safeguards

Before delving into the subject of safeguards, it may be helpful to look at how safety standards come about. While the demand for such measures may be overwhelming, initiatives are rarely introduced solely based on an adequate demonstration of their value. Hazard may be evident to many, along with the need for protective measures; yet rarely is there an immediate, wholesale adoption of safer practices. More frequently, safeguards become routine practice when exigent circumstances intersect with a certain threshold of focused concern, which is often facilitated by media attention.

An illustration is the virus responsible for HIV and the AIDS epidemic, which received center stage only after the loss of human life reached a certain crescendo in developed countries, particularly the United States. The toll on humanity, while devastating, did not serve to usher in an immediate response, despite the risk. Safety methods regarding sexual contact did not receive swift societal acceptance and compliance, even though the danger was evident. Rather, the forward propulsion in safer practices was fueled largely by a mass media campaign, which was further propelled by booster rockets powered by celebrities who championed the cause.

Certainly, we are in an age when there is no scarcity of pressing issues, throughout the world or in our country or neighborhoods. Regardless of who we are, what we do, or where we work, the issue of healthcare delivery, quality and affordability is front and center in many minds. The entire health system is intricately linked with our productivity, as a nation and as individuals. Indeed, the efficiency, quality and fiscal integrity of this industry is entwined with the economic and overall health of Wall Street, Main Street and every household.

Whether the present paradigm remains untouched or is reformed, either totally or in part, the backbone of the structure will remain intact. Regardless of any possible change to the status quo, nurses will continue to represent most of the vertebrae, as well as the heart, of healthcare.

While the patient may still wait, at times with baited breath, for the arrival of their attending physician, by and large, it is the nurse who will stay in attendance throughout each day and every night. When advocacy is called for on behalf of public health, it is the nurse's voice which will frequently intercede with legislators, insurance carriers, dietitians, physical and occupational therapists, x-ray and lab technicians. While doctors continue to write the orders, it will fall on the shoulders of nurses to actually carry them out or see to it that they are properly fulfilled. If circumstances indicate sudden or potential menace to young, old or in between, it will most often be the nurse who steps in to avert any threat. Discharge orders may be scripted, but without the nurse's keen eye to interpret the hieroglyphics, subsequent arrangements for an optimal homecoming may be overlooked.

Preserving the optimal strength, safety and dexterity of all nurses' hands is vital to every healthcare organization's ability to adequately deliver services. Every initiative which supports the discovery and implementation of optimal safeguards to protect nurses, cultivates and secures the health and safety of all.

In the United States alone, the total number of licensed nurses reaches well into the millions. The number of registered nurses is estimated at approximately two million nine hundred thousand, according to the American Nurses Association. This statistic does not include licensed practical nurses or licensed vocational nurses, which add hundreds of thousands more to this figure.

It is generally accepted that approximately ninety percent of this aggregate will not become chemically dependent in their lifetime. This vast majority of nurses will have successful, fulfilling careers, spanning decades without an untoward event, providing state-of-the-art care to the public. Routine nursing duties will continue to be performed by this overwhelming majority, including the frequent administration of controlled substances, without incident.

In spite of the predominant number of unaffected nurses, those who become chemically dependent are of grave concern to colleagues, employers and society as a whole. While those who develop a problem are certainly in the minority, due to the sheer number in the profession, the sum total of chemically dependent nurses in the United States reaches into the hundreds of thousands.

The implications become even more staggering, however, when factoring in the nursing shortage, which has prompted aggressive recruitment into the profession. Moreover, the U.S. Bureau of Labor Statistics Occupational Handbook of 2008 predicts that more than six hundred fifty thousand additional jobs will be created for RNs and LPNs between the years of 2006 and 2016.

Therefore, as the risk of chemical dependency in nursing persists, the forecast of a steep hike in existing jobs over the next decade serves to offer grim warning of an escalating storm approaching. Similar to the need for a concerted effort fostering safer sex practices to shield the public from HIV exposure, there is a looming need on the horizon to develop safeguards protecting nurses from becoming chemically dependent.

Our country is not alone in this predicament. The issue is widespread throughout the globe. No blockades exist, regardless of any military presence to secure a nation's borders. Oceans of water do not serve as effective moats, defending any country from this dilemma.

Efforts aimed at the identification of traits already apparent in the chemically dependent nurse are widespread, here and abroad. However, this is only one of the necessary steps which must be taken. The next rung in the ladder towards maximal safety is to incorporate modifications in personal behavior and professional practice which identify hazard promptly and minimize its potency whenever possible.

Increased indicators in a nurse's risk profile should be treated as seriously as nurses handle an elevation in a patient's body temperature. Thus, proactive measures may protect a nurse from harm, possibly decreasing the likelihood of acquiring a chemical dependency. Akin to monitoring a patient for signs of a fever, routine self-survey by each nurse for a heightened risk of chemical dependency may lead to timely and effective actions designed to thwart the development of a problem.

What is germane to this topic is the fundamental understanding that each and every nurse is, to some degree, vulnerable to becoming chemically dependent. The fact that most nurses escape this trap unharmed should not be confused with the illusion that one is exempt from the possibility of succumbing to this danger. Like many disease processes, chemical dependency can seize opportunistically on individuals who believe they have exceptional qualities which act as a barrier, offering immunity. As many nurses can attest, there is nothing further from the truth.

This occupational exposure is not new to nursing, nor is it unique solely to our profession. One of the most sobering facts, however, is that serious consideration has been given to this matter from within as well as outside our ranks, with only a limited impact. To date, the central focus of attention has rested predominantly on identifying and responding to those afflicted. While grappling with the predicament of those nurses already dependent on substances, less attention has been given to enhancing the security of those currently without an issue.

A more proactive approach is essential in order to identify risk markers before the appearance of an untoward event. With enlightenment regarding every nurse's professional and personal susceptibility to chemical dependency, a safety net may be cast, potentially capturing some nurses prior to a negative occurrence. Ongoing monitoring for the traits often observed in chemically dependent nurses may prompt the launching of modifications in lifestyle which may limit the exposure some may have.

The adoption of early and ongoing self-survey of nurses offers simultaneous opportunities across the spectrum of the profession. It is a means by which nursing students may be given the ability to identify issues prior to entry into the profession and the workplace. It may preempt peril with strategies which provide additional support to recently licensed nurses, who may otherwise falter during their initial transition into practice.

Those who have worked for decades, with no visible warning signs of an impending difficulty may discover a lapse in self-nurturing behavior and perform a prompt about-face. Increased stress, such as dealing with an empty nest or upcoming retirement, may be anticipated, with a plan to augment supports preemptively. Whether risk factors are insidious or sudden, the practice of ongoing self-appraisal may be successful in prompting counter-measures, which preserve the delicate balance of health and well-being.

The characteristics in the SHUNT Survey For Nurses will serve as a reference point for exploring optimal safeguards against chemical dependency. Ongoing development of proactive methods which effectively counteract these traits can offer an advantage to all nurses and the public. Though some factors may be unavoidable, the recognition of their ominous presence may afford an opportunity to mitigate any potential liability. In this manner, nurses can be safer throughout their career and lifespan.

The first "S" trait is associated with social withdrawal and self-isolative behavior. Human beings have always been referred to as social animals. Though we no longer face an urgent need to band together in large clusters to remain safe from dinosaurs and natural predators of centuries past, we continue to form groups. We share various activities of daily life with families based on blood, and communities based on where we reside. We develop workgroups based on common goals, and form religions based on spiritual beliefs. We belong to gyms to keep our waistlines trim, while eyeballing the fitness status of fellow members. We join adult education classes and athletic teams, to learn to play, or play to win any assortment of skills and sports. And when youth escapes us, sloth overtakes us, or injuries sideline us, we congregate around the television screen, giving boisterous voice to the internal critic, preferably in the company of others. From sewing circles to weekly card games, our world revolves around groups of people and our connections to those people.

Technological advances have decreased the absolute requirement for relating directly with others. No longer required to go to the market in many urban areas, email or phone orders to stock our refrigerators and pantries can now be placed. Many businesses have decided to allow employees to work one or more days per week from home.

Seminars which were once held in hotels with attendees dressed in business attire are giving way to webinars, where each person sits in the comfort of their own abode, in less restrictive fashion.

While some may have a greater tolerance for solitary pursuits, we all have occasions when socialization is anticipated. If certain company is not enjoyed, at least most of it is, more or less, endured with civility. As much as misery may love company, one's customary definition of a party is a function done collectively. But, with increased dependence on mood-altering substances comes the likelihood that this interaction with chemicals will trump all engagements with people and activities. Even contacts affording the most pleasant companionship of longstanding duration are jettisoned, in favor of mood-altering chemicals. Sacred rituals with trusted confidantes who have access to our deepest thoughts and feelings are preempted by the use of alcohol, drugs or both. Commitments which were once the very fabric of existence become displaced and eventually discarded. While the presence of this indicator may not be readily apparent to the chemically dependent nurse, it can become a bone of contention, easily recognized by those unaccustomed to their new seats on the bleachers of periphery.

The solution is to keep a well-rounded life, with multiple sources of fulfillment and many nurturing relationships. Naturally, these activities and affiliations should not revolve around substances. Remaining vigilant regarding any tendency towards life shrinkage, which is the elimination of several routine social activities and sources of support, is also beneficial.

Being able to listen with an open mind to trusted family members, friends and co-workers, who may verbalize concern over a change in attitude or behavior, may be helpful for some nurses. But confrontation by loved ones who are worried about a nurse may not be accepted at face value. A nurse may be more receptive to the concerns of family and friends if several individuals approach the nurse simultaneously. A collective group of caring individuals, who express their feelings early on, may be more difficult for a nurse to ignore. Under some circumstances, obtaining guidance from a professional with expertise in chemical dependency interventions may be appropriate.

The second "S" category, self-care behaviors beneath societal, professional or the nurse's own standards, telegraphs overlooked obligations to one's own needs. As we grow from infancy through childhood, on into adulthood, the maturation process grants us an increasing ability to care for ourselves, and eventually others. This capacity is a prerequisite for acceptance into any profession. After educational and clinical training requirements for licensure are met, there is an ongoing need for optimal functioning on a physical, emotional and professional level. This permits the laser-like concentration, emotional balance and physical stamina which is necessary to accomplish the tasks at hand.

No matter how far we advance in our expertise as nurses, we never outgrow our bodily needs for basic maintenance and self-nurturing. We are never free of our daily requirement for attentive self-care, regardless of our personal, educational or professional accomplishments. The quest for food, rest, sunlight, recreation, hygiene and other healthy customs persists. In fact, some may successfully argue that the more lofty our endeavors, and the more strenuous our efforts, the more critical are our needs for replenishment.

The cushion of safety to be interjected which alleviates the threat imposed by the second "S" trait is for nurses to care for themselves just as meticulously as they care for others. The safety instructions airline personnel recite redundantly directing us to secure our own oxygen masks prior to that of our most beloved children are apropos here.

The first "H" attribute, a family history of chemical dependency, is the hand genetics has dealt. Like it or not, this is a circumstance foisted on some, for better or worse. While a positive family history of chemical dependency poses a risk, this information can be used to great advantage. The choice to minimize or eliminate exposure to alcohol and other substances may be wise, if not crucial for some. Foregoing all consumption may be most beneficial for those whose genetic predisposition is accompanied by other indicators of risk. The operative word here, of course, is "choice." Far too many nurses come to realize, albeit too late, that had they opted to eliminate alcohol and drug use early on, they would have ultimately gained far greater freedom of choice down the road.

This also holds true for nurses with the second "H" characteristic, a history of negative consequences directly or indirectly related to their substance use. Here, the decision may be somewhat clearer. The nurse may have no residual vestige of doubt regarding the judicious course of ceasing alcohol and drug use entirely. The aftermath of such consumption may already have been painfully shocking to the nurse. Perhaps, consequences were sufficiently severe to extinguish any lingering doubt regarding the advisability of abstaining from all substances. Thus, the occurrence of disturbing events due to chemical use may have provoked positive lifestyle changes.

In cases such as these, there may be strong internal motivation for the nurse to remain clean and sober, without any pressure from outside forces. Some, however, may require additional impetus in the form of leverage, from one or more stakeholders. The intervention of family, employer, treatment provider or regulatory agency may be a necessary component for some nurses to eliminate all use.

The selection of the word "eliminate" in the preceding paragraph was quite deliberate. Once present, the second "H" indicator will never be equated as a non-existent risk factor. Regardless of how much time may pass without undesirable repercussions, a prior history of negative outcomes related to substance use is highly significant. The elimination of all mood-altering substances, unless specifically ordered by a doctor, is one safeguard which can decrease the likelihood of future heartache.

It is with firm conviction, based on education and professional experience in addiction nursing that while chemical dependency is highly responsive to optimal treatment, it is, nevertheless, a progressive condition. For many nurses with a negative experience related to chemical dependency, continued use tends to cause further untoward events. Therefore, eliminating all use, before additional repercussions occur, is one of the most effective steps any nurse can take in minimizing future risk related to this characteristic.

While individuals with a history of negative outcomes may sometimes try by various methods to moderate subsequent chemical use, this attempt often serves as further demonstration of chemical dependency's tight grasp. Rather than the nurse having the upper hand, he or she has often been subtly wooed into a feeling of personal strength. Frequently, however, quite the opposite is true. Indeed, if there is any omnipotence to be found, it is usually the substance that has staked a solid claim to it.

Regardless of technological and medical advances, there is no method available to exchange a family predisposition for a more resilient genetic make-up. Nor can we undo a mistake, even if it was done a millisecond ago. Yet, while we are all stuck with our own various ancestors and an equally unique arrangement of past faux-pas, every nurse can lay a safer foundation, in order to more adequately secure their footsteps going forward. Accepting the significance of having been dealt a hand holding either or both of the "H" indicators, gives one the opportunity to eliminate further unnecessary exposure.

Full disclosure of any family or personal history of chemical dependency to all healthcare providers is another safety measure available to every nurse. All caregivers with any capacity to order medication should receive such notification. Most qualified professionals appreciate, and even welcome, candor in this regard. Divulging this information early and fully fosters the provider's ability to determine if alternative treatments or medications may be preferable.

To exclude details when providing information to a caregiver is a risky proposition. Frequently, it leaves a door open which may become the nurse's exit ramp to a prescription drug problem. This list of providers with a need-to-know includes dentists, who frequently order pain medication. The inclination not to give due notice might be accurately perceived as resistance to a readily available safety device. Such a lack of disclosure may be regarded as a nurse exhibiting a feeling of exemption from standard protocols. Either way, this speaks volumes about the nurse's potential chance of becoming chemically dependent.

As nurses, we realize that complete and accurate historical accounts given by patients and relatives are vital components which help us render the best possible care. If our patients are less than forthcoming in their responses, we may feel somewhat short-changed. This may cause us to question subsequent information and have a measure of distrust with details already furnished. Sometimes, we may even be upset, justifiably concerned that the patient's life and our license to practice has been placed in possible jeopardy with erroneous or incomplete information.

By adhering to the customary standard of full disclosure to our own caregivers, we act the way we encourage our own patients to behave. We conform to what we regard as the prerequisite to any nurse-patient relationship: mutual trust that communication is thorough and honest. Regardless of our expertise as nurses, we do require treatment from time to time. While we may possess exceptional professional skills, our licenses do not qualify us to take any shortcuts. We are afforded no exemptions when seeking our own healthcare. So, while repetitious performance of one's professional role may produce the quintessential caregiver, the practice of being the patient, when one is the recipient of care, maintains optimal nurse safety.

The first "U" trait, untreated or unremitting emotional or physical pain, should not be ignored. Nurses can raise their level of safety and overall health by seeking timely treatment for conditions which do not respond to benign neglect. Otherwise known as lack of attention, the common cold typifies a condition that responds well to the principle of benign neglect. Thus, cold symptoms usually resolve with rest, fluids and the passage of time. The ailment is generally self-limiting, regardless of whether we lavish it with undivided attention or distract ourselves with crosswords and videos. Signs of it pass in their own time, not ours. Likewise, many other minor aches and conditions may require nothing more than rest, aspirin, fluids and patience.

However, symptoms which persist beyond a few days' duration warrant more than a wait-and-see approach. Whether a condition can be easily explained or has an undetermined cause, any significant discomfort or change in status should not have to beg our attention for very long. Nurses, like the general public, should obtain professional evaluation and treatment, sooner rather than later.

As already noted, nurses are sometimes disinclined to seek care, particularly when they estimate that their self-management of symptoms is possible or preferable. Sometimes a longstanding issue is a source of great embarrassment which further delays scheduling an appointment with a qualified practitioner. This can occur with physical as well as emotional symptoms. While a postponement might not be lethal, it does nothing to safeguard the nurse.

Ongoing dialogue with caregivers can be extremely beneficial, not just for our patients, but for ourselves as well. Advocating with our own providers in the midst of not feeling well is certainly very difficult at times. Yet, it remains essential for us to impart information back to the practitioner, particularly if the prescribed treatment falls short of providing adequate remedy.

In cases where the nurse's symptoms endure and energies are being depleted, the nurse should seek the support of trusted colleagues, friends or family members to assist in the advocacy process. Requesting such assistance early in the course of treatment may be desirable, particularly if symptoms are likely to be prolonged or very taxing.

The second "U" characteristic can be kept at bay by taking medications exactly as prescribed by one's provider. Nurses who determine their own off-label use are entering dangerous territory. This includes not mixing medications with alcohol or other substances, which may alter the effect of the prescription. Once again, it is vital to maintain an ongoing dialogue with providers regarding any matters of concern. If there are side effects, or a desire to cease the medication entirely, the subject should be discussed with the caregiver before altering any of the prescribed treatment. If several professionals are rendering care simultaneously, all should have waivers permitting disclosure to each other. Such conferences may be essential to ensure well-coordinated care as well as optimal nurse safety.

Before offering any methods of protection against the first "N" characteristic, nursing practice routinely in excess of fifty-five hours per week, emphasis must be placed on this category's linchpin quality. While all SHUNT indicators are separate attributes, excessive work as a nurse has a knack for innervating the participation of several other risk factors. This can occur in rapid, almost simultaneous fashion. Therefore, this trait is of pivotal importance, because interwoven within it are catalytic threads which may automatically enervate other elements of risk to an activated state.

This domino effect is seen when excessive work hours eliminate the opportunity to spend our time and energy elsewhere. Social gatherings may be precluded, as well as exercise and dental care, introducing the first and second "S" categories into the mix.

Overwork may camouflage signs of depression or bully symptoms of pain into submission. Pushed from view, the seeds of discomfort and distress may go untreated. This may sometimes lead to self-medicating behaviors, ushering in the first or second "U" factor, or both.

Another scenario caused by an excessive number of hours working as a nurse may be sparked by turmoil, when spouse or children feel neglected. This can increase a nurse's stress, particularly if any objections voiced are accompanied by a lack of cooperation. A corresponding lack of assistance with household chores by one or more family members is not unusual in such instances. Sometimes children express their discontent by not fulfilling homework assignments or by paying less attention to grades which may plummet.

So, nurses working in excess of fifty-five hours per week, month after month, have less time available for socialization, rest, recreation and general attention to self-nurturing behaviors. This adds tension to an already pressured lifestyle. All of these variables enter into the equation, eroding one's resilience and resistance to illness and injury. Vulnerability to chemical dependency is just one of the possible repercussions. Additionally, there may be miscalculations in judgment when caring for patients. In an environment where any errors may lead to patient harm, a devastating result may occur, impacting the patient as well as the nurse. The possible outcome of any error may very well have a serious ripple effect on the nurse's professional license to practice.

A preponderance of studies has yielded a firm correlation between the number of hours nurses worked beyond a customary eight-hour shift and the amount of mistakes they made. The evidence has been so compelling that it has prompted some states to enact legislation banning employers from mandating nurses to work overtime.

The full-time equivalent of most nursing positions is roughly forty hours per week. This is exclusive of any commute to and from work. There is no question that the demands of most nursing jobs are extreme, not just physically and intellectually, but emotionally. Routinely working hours in a nursing capacity which are significantly above the full-time complement designated for that position should only be done after much soul searching.

Nurses should pause long enough to consider their current risk profile, in its entirety, before diving head-first into this potential firestorm which poses so much potential downside. Mindfulness to the length and the quality of round-trip commute, childcare duties, and other responsibilities which may not be readily delegated to others, should be taken into account. These variables should then be factored into each nurse's unique profile of risk.

Routinely working less than fifty-five hours per week provides greater opportunity for balance between the professional and personal facets of life. This promotion of a healthy lifestyle supports wellness and enables wholesome habits, which can minimize stress. Additionally, moderate work schedules can keep a number of other traits from partnering with the excessive work factor, thus minimizing adverse situations.

The second "N" factor, nursing duties include
frequent access to controlled substances, is a
characteristic which accompanies a majority of
traditional nursing roles. In some positions, it is
not just one of several essential tasks, but the core
of duties the nurse is responsible for. While most
drugs manufactured are not habit-forming, there
are some which are particularly problematic.
These preparations have prompted heightened
safety concerns, due to their propensity to being
abused. Collectively categorized as "controlled
substances," this term signifies that attempts have
been made to regulate and control their use. Thus,
these drugs require special procedures related to
prescribing, handling and administering them.

Frequent access to these habit-forming substances
has long been a recognized occupational hazard in
nursing. While the vast majority of nurses do not
succumb to any temptation, some nurses do
become dependent on these drugs and procure
them from the workplace. As previously noted,
this process of illegally obtaining substances from
the employer is known as drug diversion.

Most nurses have a fundamental belief that they are
incapable of such actions. Nursing students never
imagine as they embark upon their career that they
will ever steal drugs from employers. More

seasoned nurses have an equally unshakeable belief that drug diversion will never be an option considered, let alone taken.

Therefore, any problem with controlled substances usually begins insidiously without fanfare, and in shadows which are hidden from view. Sometimes in hindsight, a chemically dependent nurse is able to trace the advent of an issue back to a combination of precipitant factors.

One of the most familiar experiences is having had a previous prescription for dental work or another legitimate medical necessity. In some instances, nurses have remarked to their physicians that the particular habit-forming substance ordered actually lifted their mood. For those who have any history of depression which has required antidepressant medication, this effect of mood-altering substances may be problematic. This is especially pertinent if previously prescribed interventions have proven ineffective in relieving symptoms.

Other nurses have cited that mood-altering substances made them feel normal or better able to cope with stressors. Whatever feeling may be elicited, however, some of these legitimate prescriptions do open the gates to a subsequent craving. Regardless of where the medication is obtained, continued use may develop into chemical dependency. As inadvertently and unintentionally as this progression from use to dependence may have begun, some cases have resulted in premeditated and intentional acts of drug diversion in the workplace.

Employers and regulatory agencies have attempted to address the grave situation of drug diversion in numerous ways. The ultimate goal, of course, is to eliminate the illegal procurement of medications from the work site. Some innovations have met with relative success, thus making diversion of substances more difficult to accomplish. These measures, coupled with insightful audits by pharmacy and oversight from others, have led to more timely detection of drug diversion in many cases.

Various systems have been designed in order to offer greater assurance that controlled substances are not tampered with. Regulatory agencies have established protocols to ensure that medications traverse a direct path from the manufacturer to the intended recipient, without detour, substitution or dilution. Technological advances have also been implemented which feature elaborate safety mechanisms to prevent theft of drugs. Computerized systems with PIN codes which identify the nurse responsible for dispensing the medication have been employed in many institutions and offer enhanced security. However, no system has yet been able to claim one hundred percent effectiveness in totally eliminating diversion of medication from the workplace.

Regardless of the protocol used, several practices can raise the level of safety for all nurses. The first is related to the procedures used to waste medications. When an order is written for a dose which is not available in the exact amount ordered, some of the medication must be wasted. If the medication is a controlled substance, special policies are in place to ensure that the excess amount is, indeed, wasted.

Regulations generally require that another nurse must witness this process of wasting any medication which is identified as a controlled substance. The nurse providing witness must sign his or her name alongside that of the colleague administering the medication. While affixing a signature to a document takes no more than a few seconds, there is much more involved in executing this procedure properly.

In order to fulfill the role of witness completely, the nurse is obligated to be present and in observance of the entire process. Technically, the witness is verifying, with his or her signature, that the medication was found intact, with the manufacturer's seal unbroken; that the seal was broken under their watchful eye; that they saw the ordered amount set aside for the patient; and that the remainder, the portion to be wasted, was properly disposed of, also in their sight. When performed with precision, this procedure takes at least two or more minutes, depending upon whether the medication to be given is a pill or an injection.

A few minutes, versus seconds, is only a matter of several extra breaths and a few dozen blinks of the eye. As inconsequential as this time may seem, when multiplying these few extra minutes by the number of times that medications are unavailable in the exact dosage ordered, the total mounts quickly to well beyond a few minutes. Those few minutes must then be multiplied by two in each case of witnessing a waste, because when fully executed this process requires the concentrated focus of not just one, but two pairs of eyes.

Thus, following this procedure, by the book, becomes much more demanding on available nursing resources than a mere signature would be. In a job where minutes and seconds are sometimes the only line dividing life, death and near-miss experiences, the temptation to forego all or part of the proper waste protocol is enormous.

The perception in many nurses' minds, which is sometimes given voice to, is that witnessing medication waste is wasting time. Add to this the fact that most nurses view their co-workers, at the very least, with a modicum of trust and respect. This tends to place the nurse performing the waste, and the nurse witnessing it, in a tug-of-war, in which both are struggling with the following dilemma: Just how does one go about insisting on a repetitive, redundant fulfillment of procedure, without insulting one's fellow nurse? To wit, the reply is: The proper execution of witnessing a waste is either done in full or not at all.

To affix one's signature to the medication record, which is a legal document, when the complete protocol is not followed is fraud. This falsification of records can result in prosecution, criminally and/or professionally. The culmination of any charges may be that a nurse's license sits precariously in the scales of justice, rather than in a frame on wall or desk.

So, a more pertinent question a nurse might ask would be: Is the time, money and effort spent in obtaining my nursing license which affords me the privilege to practice my profession of greater value than saving a few minutes by skimping on proper execution of a task I am legally obligated to perform? Does fulfilling my professional and legal obligations and maintaining my license in good standing rank above the feelings of any colleague? For most nurses who have ever asked themselves these questions, there is little need for contemplation, prior to responding.

Another safeguard related to the handling of controlled substances is the strict enforcement by employers of the standards which have been set for witnessing the waste of medications. In many facilities, these policies are reviewed regularly and as situations may arise. All facilities should hold all nurses accountable for following these procedures, to the letter, as these standards offer one of the greatest protective mechanisms regarding exposure to the second "N" trait.

Sometimes, issues become apparent to staff nurses long before supervisors and policymakers. As nurses go about their tasks, they frequently encounter situations which may not be visible at other levels of the organization. Solutions may also be evident to nurses, as well as those in other professions within the healthcare system.

Most administrators would agree that the devil truly is in the details, especially when trying to formulate best practices. Some have enlisted the input of employees throughout their institution, by establishing anonymous drop boxes for employee suggestions and issues of concern. In this way, problems apparent on any level of the organization may be aired which may have otherwise been lost to policymakers. Proposed solutions may also come to the surface in this manner.

Many healthcare administrators have taken steps to foster communication up the chain and between departments. In this way, different perspectives can be shared. Better understanding of each department's role, and the challenges entailed in fulfilling those tasks, is extremely important in obtaining cooperation between functional units.

Without even knowing it, some non-nursing employees may play a role in safety related to controlled substances. One such example may be the housekeeping department, which is often responsible for ensuring that the refuse bins are emptied regularly. Sometimes, housekeeping staff may not be aware of the possible hazard to nurses when the overflowing receptacle happens to be the box which needles are deposited in. In some units, this may also be the container into which nurses deposit the remnants of controlled substance vials and syringes. Thus, any materials which fall partially outside a full bin may be taken.

Continuous education for all nursing staff, which focuses on safeguards as well as the importance of following the facility's protocols, should be offered. Additionally, annual classes should be mandatory regarding the inherent risk of chemical dependency in the profession. As many other departments often interact closely with nurses, individuals from these areas should also be periodically reminded of the hazards which exist in the workplace. Every employee should be well-versed in the steps which should be taken in the event suspicious behavior is observed in a nurse or other individual.

Employers sometimes solicit input from the facility's legal counsel in formulating protocols which should be followed in the event questionable circumstances arise regarding an employee's actions or appearance. As there are many federal, state and other statutory codes which may be applicable, depending on the type of facility and the classification of patient, these matters often become quite complex. Navigating through this terrain, where circumstances may be unclear, often requires the advice of several experts. Depending on the circumstances, opinions may be sought from those knowledgeable in regulatory statutes, employment issues, chemical dependency and the nursing profession.

Regardless of the degree of clarity or murkiness, however, it is imperative for employers to take appropriate action. Offering a benign reference to any nurse suspected of drug diversion in lieu of termination, instead of making a report to the necessary agency, is never a wise or ethical approach. Such administrative decisions only serve to pass the suspected nurse on to another facility, where problems may escalate, causing greater chance of harm to the public and the nurse.

A safety mechanism for the first "T" factor, a transitional period requiring major adjustment within the past year, is to modulate the volume of change which occurs over a brief interval, whenever possible. Events which are volitional in nature can sometimes be staggered along an extended, rather than abrupt, timeline.

Often, an impending marriage is in the planning stages for many months, if not years, permitting one to more gradually introduce other requisite changes, such as relocating to a new residence. Changing employment due to the nuptials may be initiated with due thought given to the overall landscape of change already underway. Careful deliberation may spur a decision to delay some of the concurrent adjustments, until a quieter interval in life.

One of the most cherished highlights in life, the birth of a child, is also one of the most challenging experiences. This celebrated event frequently sparks several lifestyle modifications, such as the relocation to a larger home, and obligatory alterations in finances, priorities, schedule, leisure activities and sleep habits.

Certainly, separation and divorce are huge transitional periods, often necessitating a change in living arrangements, money matters and social contacts. Again, due care should be used in making these changes, to take full advantage of any opportunities to stagger the required adjustments.

Some transitional events are on the radar for decades, such as a child leaving for college or getting married. The first child to make their exit may not be felt as acutely as the second or last. Empty nests often seem to arrive at the peak of other life-changing events, such as menopause, or the declining health or death of a parent.

Probably no transition has been longer anticipated than the arrival of our so-called golden years. The eons spent eagerly looking forward to our ability to answer to no one, especially the alarm clock, often holds one enraptured, sometimes for decades. Lulled by dreams spun by advertisers of smooth sailing, we may miss the buoys of reality which may alert us to the rough waves ahead. After arrival of these long-awaited years, often portrayed as brimming with freedom and happiness in slick and shiny advertisements, one may find this stage lacks the jutting rocks one often clung to during times of stress.

The absence of purpose and connectivity which working and interacting with colleagues afforded us is lost. The addition of much free time is usually accompanied by a fair share of the aches of aging. As such, this era may very well be one of the most underestimated in terms of obstacles to be faced. In spite of any and all financial preparations we may have made, we may find ourselves psychologically and physically challenged, as well as possibly unprepared.

Every transition cannot be planned for, of course. Sudden and sometimes unpleasant changes are often unavoidable. In spite of that, there may be the ability to interject protective elements which create a zone of safety. Using some of the SHUNT factors as a guide, a nurse may chart a course for navigating around, rather than through, at least some of the tropical storms of transitional periods.

Increasing the quality and frequency of time spent with key supportive people, such as relatives, friends and colleagues, may provide familiarity which improves one's ability to cope with change. Greater attention to self-care and nurturing through activities, such as long walks, listening to music, reading, journaling or working on creative projects, may provide healthy outlets.

Utilizing accrued time off, instead of excessive hours at work, may be beneficial and protective of one's resources. The awareness that all change, whether desired or dreaded, requires a period of adjustment may provoke one to be kinder and gentler in their expectations of self.

While some may persist in the belief that the person who hesitates is apt to be lost, being respectfully cautious regarding the total amount of hurdles one tackles at a time can be of great benefit. Careful attention in this regard definitely affords nurses an additional safeguard that should be taken. Recognition with acceptance of the rippling impact change can exert on anyone's life is, in itself, a safeguard. But, regardless of transformation underway, it is essential not to summarily dismiss it, without ascertaining its potential effect.

Turmoil or tragedy with unresolved conflict, the second "T" factor, is a part of human existence no one escapes entirely. Like a poker hand, it is not the cards of turmoil or tragedy so much as what we do with them that counts.

While tragedy is often sudden, unexpected and unwelcome, it is also usually of such magnitude that it cannot be denied for long. Often, it successfully claims our undivided attention, as well as that of the people around us. This sets the stage for commencing the process of resolution. Though there may be several steps involved in dealing fully with grief or loss, tragedy undoubtedly makes its presence known in a manner which invokes that journey.

The coping methods we use may depend largely on the situation, as well as our past experience, level of functioning and available supports. Death of a loved one, serious injury, catastrophic fire or weather-related disaster which destroys a home, are all examples of tragic circumstances. While we may not have the tight-knit communities we had several generations ago, there are often people who rally to our side during these times of crises.

Although we may be reluctant to accept help, we may give in, acquiescing at a point just shy of being totally overwhelmed. Even if circumstances do not push us to the brink, the offers graciously made do, at the very least, bring the solace and comfort of knowing we have merited some attention. This reminder, that someone cares, is important in and of itself. We are, therefore, not left feeling completely unnoticed, alone and bereft.

While turmoil may be a much less daunting prospect than tragedy, it is also less likely to get our attention or that of others. Rather than reconciling the issue which provoked it, turmoil may be readily dismissed, and more easily ignored. An example may be the nurse who has gone to work with the often familiar knot of conflict and anxiety over leaving young children in the care of others. In another instance, it may be that of the nurse who stays in an emotionally abusive relationship because there is no actual physical abuse.

In the absence of escalating circumstances, resolution may not occur. In spite of the situation being troublesome and stressful, the ongoing conflict may be allowed to continue, albeit at a price. The act of repeatedly swallowing what one finds unacceptable often exacts a toll. For some, the stress relief provided by mood-altering substances permits maintaining the status quo of turmoil one may find difficult or almost intolerable to live with.

The choice for some may be to avail themselves of support groups, specifically designed to deal with parental, marital or other issues. Some may seek the expertise of a qualified therapist or counselor. A combination of using both support groups and individual counseling may be an option enlisted by others. Methods which assist one in developing short-term strategies and better coping skills have been helpful to many.

While the safeguards listed in this chapter may be a guide in averting some nurses from becoming chemically dependent, it is probable that a fair number may go on to develop an issue. It is also likely that some nurses will progress in their chemical dependency to a point when untoward or even near catastrophic events may be encountered

The next chapter details some of the troubling events which have occurred when a nurse's chemical dependency has progressed. In most of

Chapter 4: Optimal Safeguards

these situations, nurses did not have full comprehension of the tenacity and virulence of their condition; nor did they have any accurate estimation of the amount of outside help they needed.

Sentinel Events

I am sitting at the window of a twenty-fourth floor hotel room in Manhattan, after concluding some business related to publishing this book. The vehicles below remind me of the Matchbox cars I once loved as a child. Life was very simple then, cut and dried. Societal values were vastly different and families, more often than not, had dinner together.

Life was by no means idyllic. There were harsh reminders of reality and how fragile and precious each breath truly is. The natural order was that the elderly grandparent would become less able to successfully catch a wayward child. Odds were that youth would be permitted transit to that very same era of declining abilities, albeit with improved wisdom and insight. With advancing age comes mounting awareness that when we have our health, we are in possession of the greatest treasure on earth.

The highest level of health and functioning, however, is not a reality for the chemically dependent nurse, especially after a sentinel event. The Joint Commission on the Accreditation of Healthcare Organizations, or JCAHO, which accredits hospitals in the United States, has defined a sentinel event as "an unexpected occurrence involving death or serious physical or psychological injury or the risk thereof." The JCAHO goes on to explain the meaning of the phrase "or the risk thereof" as including "any process variation, for which a recurrence would carry a significant chance of a serious adverse outcome."

Due to nursing's pivotal role in healthcare delivery, patients are greatly impacted by the overall health of every nurse. Though far from exhaustive, the following examples may help one in identifying sentinel events which may be related to chemical dependency in some nurses. Recognizing these situations may lead to more timely intervention, thus forwarding the goals of the Joint Commission, as well as the healthcare industry and the nursing profession.

One of the most noticeable situations is a nurse arriving at work with alcohol on their breath, or other signs of being under the influence. The cause of impairment may be due to a legitimate prescription and/or the use of a recreational drug. Regardless of the causative agent, however, once a nurse's condition is observed as less than optimal, actions must be taken immediately. Employers are usually swift to respond in such cases by relieving the nurse of professional duties.

This occasion, however, calls for more than sheer removal of the nurse from the workplace. There is a responsibility far beyond calling for a brief time-out from patient care. The nurse should ideally be leveraged into having a mandatory evaluation by a competent and objective third party. In this way, the nurse may be directed to treatment, if indicated.

In addition to eliminating the nurse's contact with patients, pre-established state reporting protocols must be met. Such requirements usually demand the submission of documentation, noting specific details regarding the incident. While some facilities may prefer not to render such formal notification, nonconformance with regulations is fraught with hazards.

This peril extends not just to the nurse and the employer, but to patients. While some institutions may believe that the chemically dependent nurse can be spared unnecessary anguish if such a matter is handled in-house, this decision generally reaps diminished results, and sometimes havoc, for all involved. Actions which circumvent any reporting policy established by a state compromise the nurse's recovery, as well as the needs of patients and the facility.

The rationale for non-compliance with regulatory directives may be concern that less than optimal practices at the facility may be exposed by any ensuing investigation. There may be some apprehension related to adequate staffing levels. Maintaining the minimum number of nurses to provide proper care may be further impacted if a chemically dependent nurse is precluded from working due to report of a sentinel event.

Employers may be wary that once a regulatory agency is notified, their hands will be tied in this, as well as other matters which may come to light. While these reasons may provoke reluctance on the part of a facility to file a report, nothing overrides the more pressing priority of preventing a more significant, possibly catastrophic event.

Nurses who have executed the supreme error in judgment of reporting for duty under the influence are usually more than slightly affected by chemical use. Indiscretions of this caliber are frequently the hallmark of decreased insight and self-control. Such behavior unequivocally communicates the chemically dependent nurse's imminent need for intervention, evaluation and follow-up.

Many employers take prompt, proactive measures, reporting the chemically dependent nurse and placing them on a leave of absence in order to receive optimal treatment. Some organizations may subsequently support the nurse in a return to practice, once recovery milestones are met. Other facilities may opt, for numerous reasons, to discharge the nurse from employment. Whatever decision is reached regarding future job prospects, there is a paramount need for an impartial and qualified party to evaluate the nurse and make specific recommendations. Just as the nurse is unable to remedy the situation alone, so too is the employer unable to bring this matter to resolution, without outside assistance.

In spite of an institution's best intentions of supporting a chemically dependent nurse, the facility's primary concern is to run a business. This cardinal rule is as applicable in healthcare as in any other industry. That business is providing the best healthcare services possible to patients. Thus, when push comes to shove, as it does in every healthcare organization, the employer will have no choice, except to forego the needs of the nurse in favor of those of the patient.

As giving short shrift to the nurse ultimately meets the needs of no one if the nurse's recovery does not remain intact, it is far better that facilities focus on their business of caring for patients. The business of safeguarding the recovery of the chemically dependent staff member is better placed in the hands of more impartial parties, such as an employee assistance program or a bona fide treatment provider.

Another sentinel event related to chemical dependency which may become apparent in the workplace is discrepancies in medication records due to the diversion of drugs. Sometimes this may have begun inadvertently when a patient refused a medication which a nurse was about to administer. The nurse may have been waylaid by the needs of another patient en route back to the medication room.

As demands on nurses are frequently pressing and relentless during a shift, it may slip a nurse's mind altogether that the drug has not been returned. Thus, the matter may not have been rectified prior to the nurse leaving work at the end of the shift. The pill or syringe may have been pocketed, only to be discovered after arriving home.

At this point, the nurse must decide how to proceed. While making an immediate disclosure to the nurse's supervisor may seem to require no deliberation, this is sometimes perceived by the nurse as a more complex matter. Nurses may face some internal conflict regarding giving this notice because informing superiors of such an error usually involves more than a cursory adjustment of paperwork. Fear that the breach may lead to a reprimand, written warning, or other sanction may give the nurse reason to pause. If there have been any past issues with performance, the nurse may be even more reluctant to report the mistake. In light of the possible ramifications to continued employment, the decision may be made to keep quiet.

In this hushed environment, the facility is not informed that the medication was not given. If the secret is kept, the nurse faces another choice: to destroy the medication or save it. The story may well end here for the nurse who opts to discard the substance. But it may have only begun for the nurse who has set it aside; for inherent in this act is often a subconscious thought of future use.

Therefore, this is not an insignificant decision for any nurse. The die is often cast at this point, even though months may pass without giving this matter another thought. A very solid line of boundaries between employer and nurse has been crossed, setting the stage for the future procurement of drugs in this or a similar manner. This seed may germinate for an indeterminate length of time before use actually takes place.

At some point, though, physical or emotional discomfort may prompt the nurse to reach for this seemingly quick, innocuous fix. This act is often accompanied by the belief that this is a solution which will be utilized "just this once." What often escapes the nurse's awareness, however, is that whatever provoked this initial desire for relief is usually a circumstance or condition which is recurrent in nature.

In order to keep the workplace sacrosanct, some nurses may choose to entice a legitimate prescription from a doctor. Others may obtain their supply through internet sources. Some may take the route of stealing a prescription pad, forging an order to be filled at one or more pharmacies where they are not personally known.

Having stepped over the line once at work, however, some nurses do return to that source, setting in motion a repetitious cycle of drug diversion. Although the vast majority of nurses who divert drugs obtain them in a manner which they believe will not harm patients, actions now become deliberate. One such method is through selecting drugs which must be wasted. These are usually situations in which the ordered dose is smaller than the dosage available for distribution. Another path is a contrived maneuver, targeting patients who have medications ordered, but do not need or desire one or more of their doses. Sometimes totally fictitious names of non-existent patients may be logged in the medication record, especially in settings where there is a high turnover of cases.

Some facilities have converted to computerized systems, which require the nurse to enter their PIN code prior to obtaining a dose of medication. This allows for more efficient tracking of individual nurses, as well as patients. In some instances, however, a colleague's code may be stolen to gain access to drugs, while concealing the true identity of the nurse who actually took the substance.

Although rare, there are some nurses whose chemical dependency has progressed to the point where they have given a patient in need of medication a placebo, while pocketing the dose for their own use. This circumstance may be more apt to befall a less alert patient, in the hopes that the situation is not uncovered.

Drug manufacturers have expanded the availability of various individual dose containers over the years, reducing the need for multiple dose vials. Security measures have also been added to more readily identify tampered supplies. Though rare, some nurses have manipulated stock medications, extracting the desired substance and substituting another.

The implications of all these situations are enormous, particularly the latter ones which involve the welfare of patients and the reputation of co-workers. But there are other events, such as a nurse who falls asleep at the desk or has an altercation with a patient or staff member which are also troubling. Sometimes substance use is the underlying cause of excessive fatigue, as well as eruptions in emotion. While co-workers may become aware of such instances, they may be reluctant to report these matters up the chain of command, as per established protocol. They may feel a wall of silence is appropriate to protect a fellow worker. At times, colleagues may think that the matter is insignificant.

Particularly in cases where the observer may be under the supervision of the chemically dependent nurse, there may be fear of retribution if the whistle is blown. If facilities have established alternative protocols for these or similar situations, such procedures should be followed. One rule of thumb which remains fairly consistent in every state and setting is that one-to-one confrontations with the chemically dependent nurse should usually be avoided.

Many facilities have established somewhat formal procedures, whereby two or more key individuals confront a nurse regarding problematic or suspicious behavior. The nurse's response at the time may be one of denial of any problem. There may be rationalizations with pat excuses, such as a lack of sleep, overwork or not feeling well, which are given as the precipitant for a change in appearance or behavior. The chemically dependent nurse may lash out verbally in anger, abruptly leaving the facility. More frequently, however, the nurse admits to having a problem and expresses willingness to follow all instructions given.

Confrontation is often an overwhelming process for all involved. For the chemically dependent nurse, the combination of stress and the effects of substance use may compromise the ability to comprehend, and later recall, details that were verbally communicated. For this reason, some employers provide the nurse with a formal written document, enumerating instructions, as well as expectations.

Deadlines may be listed for the completion of certain tasks, such as contacting the employee assistance program and undergoing a chemical dependency evaluation by a treatment provider. The nurse may be provided with numbers for nurse peer support group meetings available in the area and instructed to attend. Application for enrollment into the alternative to discipline program may also be noted as mandatory. This written checklist of the nurse's responsibilities serves as a point of reference going forward, at a time when information may be initially misinterpreted, or later forgotten.

Relatives and friends may or may not be surprised when a nurse informs them that they have been placed on a leave of absence related to drug or alcohol use. Some intimate with the chemically dependent nurse may have been aware there was an issue. Particularly if the substance was obtained from work, however, loved ones may be totally blindsided

When those close to the chemically dependent nurse realize there is a problem with drugs and/or alcohol, such information is not usually shared with the employer, for obvious reasons. Many relatives and friends have a vested interest in the nurse maintaining employment. Sometimes the indicators apparent in a nurse's personal life are just as ominous as any symptoms displayed at work. When family members and friends allow recognition of such signals to slip by, without a prompt and adequate response, a valuable opportunity is lost.

Many close to a chemically dependent nurse have lived to regret their self-imposed silence. In the face of warning signs, some concerned observers have discovered that they were permitted no subsequent opportunity for an intervention, after the initial discovery of an issue. Sentinel events, unheeded, can escalate rapidly. This is especially true for nurses, who have ready access to extremely potent substances, usually in vast quantity. While many of these cases do not proceed to fatality, unfortunately, some do.

In some instances a nurse's substance use may cause a loss of consciousness. If this occurs at the workplace or in public, there is usually a swift response from bystanders. There is often little that can be said by a nurse to dissuade those present from taking aggressive steps to ensure that medical attention is rendered.

But, if this happens at the nurse's home or in their car, there may be an absence of onlookers. On occasions when family and/or friends are in attendance, a nurse may be revived, yet adamantly refuse emergency treatment. In spite of any nurse being aroused without a call to 911, the occurrence is extremely serious. While this may be the first time such an event was witnessed, it may not be the first time for such an occurrence. Thus, any occasion which leads to the discovery of a nurse in an unresponsive state should prompt observers to insist upon a thorough examination, on the spot.

Sometimes those intimate with the chemically dependent nurse find syringes, track marks or persistent bruises on the body. When these circumstances are explained easily by the nurse, but no truth resonates in the recipient's ears, these discoveries should not be dismissed. Especially when accompanied by changes in behavior or secretiveness, such evidence should never be ignored.

When cognition of the seriousness of the situation dawns, loved ones are often at a loss, not knowing where to turn. In the absence of absolute certainty as to what should be done, many begin to think they may very well be imagining things. Some start to believe they may be making too much of the situation, which will take care of itself in time. But far from being out of proportion, these perceptions may be tacitly correct. With even the barest acknowledgment of the implications, most relatives and friends become overwhelmed, if not terrified. Feelings of alarm may yield to deflation so pronounced that even the most titanic of hearts would sink. The inclination to descend into paralysis in the light of such unthinkable thoughts, however, must give way to action.

Contacting an expert professional who specializes in chemical dependency treatment has been of help to many. Often, an objective and astute professional can offer the best advice on how to proceed. Hotline numbers for dealing with issues related to chemical dependency are available in some areas. Clergy frequently have knowledge of local resources which may be able to provide assistance, support and guidance to family members and friends. If circumstances seem to dictate, a professionally orchestrated intervention may be an option for some.

The resource list at the back of this book, though far from complete, may highlight additional avenues of support and information which may be of interest and available to some. Although contact information was verified prior to publication, there is no assurance that details will remain accurate in the future.

Sentinel events are significant occurrences. The earlier they are recognized and addressed, the less likely an escalation or repetition of untoward incidents. For those who care about a chemically dependent nurse, these negative occurrences may very well be a valuable card in an otherwise lousy hand. But in order to avail oneself of the value of a sentinel event, the card must be played, rather than left on the table.

All concerned parties are stakeholders in these situations. From the employer and colleagues, to the relatives and friends, all have an investment in the well-being of the chemically dependent nurse. Separately or in tandem, all those involved can exert leverage on the nurse, often with very powerful effect.

At the time of a sentinel event, many chemically dependent nurses are willing, yet unable, to bring about a change in their lives. They often intuit that their own hand is played out, but lack the ability to stop on their own. While the desire to cease use is often strong, the chemically dependent nurse is truly powerless without the intervention of others.

Therefore, the stakeholder who has properly identified the magnitude of the situation holds the upper hand. Stepping forward with an expert's professional guidance, rather than remaining inert when faced with such a challenge, may protect a most priceless resource: a chemically dependent nurse's life.

In order to facilitate the nurse's recovery and the safety of others, however, a sabbatical from professional practice is frequently essential. The following chapter highlights this often necessary hiatus from working as a nurse.

Reprieve From Professional Practice

The occurrence of a sentinel event at the workplace is a serious matter. So too are many less prominent behavioral displays which may prompt the intervention of relatives or friends. Chemical dependency which has sparked a confrontation on a professional level often requires a leave from nursing practice. This allows the chemically dependent nurse to focus on treatment. It also unmistakably communicates the gravity of the situation to the nurse. A leave from practice also unquestionably places the chemically dependent nurse in the role of treatment recipient, rather than the provider of care.

Typically, nurses are held in very high regard by the public. It is a profession, however, which frequently necessitates one to be assertive. As nurses direct care in many settings, our role often carries an heir of authority. Therefore, we are often in a position to make a polite request or more impertinently bark out orders, as the situation warrants. From respectfully asking visitors to leave the bedside, to demanding a patient with nasal oxygen extinguish a cigarette, there is no doubt that we are viewed by others, as well as ourselves, as being in command.

However, one of the most fundamental requirements of the earliest phase of chemical dependency treatment is the ability to follow instructions, rather than dish them out. This is a challenge for many nurses, particularly when it is regarding our own health and well-being. This hurdle is often raised somewhat by a nurse's tendency to intellectualize a diagnosis of chemical dependency. After all, we know much about the subject, and its treatment. But spouting forth chapter and verse of medical and scientific facts regarding the addicted brain, neurotransmitters, and pleasure pathways is light-years away from being able to live a clean and sober life, one day at a time.

The prerequisite to any recovery from chemical dependency is a truly receptive, open mind. This receptivity is best accomplished when one dismisses what one supposes one knows, and what one thinks one is supposed to know.

Rather than a diagnosis read about in a nursing journal, it is absolutely vital for the chemically dependent nurse to own the diagnosis as a disorder they have acquired. This identification and oneness with the condition is a primary and vital ingredient in any nurse's treatment. Although in many cases this is a tall order, this acceptance places the nurse undeniably in a frame of mind which is fertile for recovery.

True acceptance of this diagnosis entails removing one's nursing cap, in favor of the hat of the chemically dependent individual who is receiving, rather than rendering and directing, treatment. More than cursory acknowledgment of this fact is paramount. While stepping out of the familiar driver's seat is difficult enough for most nurses, accepting the full implications of having a chemical dependency on a personal, gut level is an even greater leap. However, without complete integration of the attitudes and actions which correspond with full acceptance, an uninterrupted recovery may remain elusive.

For some nurses, this acceptance of their plight may come at the beginning of the treatment process. Some may experience a sentinel event of such proportions that they are almost struck into a state of submission. There is more than a cursory acquiescence to the diagnosis and demands of treatment. The identification as a nurse becomes profoundly adjusted; it becomes secondary to the identification as a chemically dependent nurse.

This changed perception in identity is a slower, sometimes arduous process for other nurses. Acceptance may come and go, in fits and starts. There may be characteristics of intermittent and superficial resignation which may appear similar to an electrical short in a wire. In these nurses, a short circuit in acceptance may blink on and off, unpredictably.

But whether the nurse is jolted into sudden acceptance, or experiences a more circuitous route to acquiring this quality, the process can be easily compromised if one remains keenly focused on conducting business as usual. And for nurses, this business is ministering to others.

Habitual thoughts and behaviors which precipitated sentinel events are often of longstanding duration. Often, these patterns have had their start much earlier in life. Although many of these habits may predate actual substance use, they may inadvertently support the re-initiation of drugs and/or alcohol use. Teasing out these sometimes intricately woven fibers is a complicated and painstaking task. Human nature, like Mother Nature, abhors a vacuum. Therefore, the mere excision of thoughts and behaviors which are incompatible with recovery would leave a void. These hollow spaces would be incapable of supporting the framework of recovery and attract a return of old, familiar patterns. Thus, detrimental thoughts, attitudes and actions must be replaced by others which optimally support recovery. Similar to the rehabilitation process for many conditions, this change takes time, focus, energy and ongoing commitment.

In the case of the chemically dependent nurse, health must take precedence, or continued professional practice is impossible. There must be continuous, astute awareness and vigilance on the part of the nurse. If treatment is shortchanged, or recovery is taken for granted, it can lead to fatality. It is unlikely that this fact can ever be burned too indelibly into a nurse's mind. When there is a substantial pause from distractions, however, a nurse has the opportunity to fully reflect on the significance of the situation. Therefore, a compelling respite from professional duties often engenders a better chance that all the implications of this diagnosis will remain fully acknowledged.

The pivotal role of a reprieve from practice is not solely due to the time which is available for recovery efforts; nor is it simply prepping the mind to an open and treatable state. Such a respite also renders a clear and constant climate, ripe for change. The time out, usually accompanied by a very noticeable loss of income, usually forces one to overhaul priorities. There is a re-examination of values, with the elimination of non-essentials. One establishes a new economy, based on necessities. Much of what was once viewed as vitally important yields, taking a more respectful position behind the nurse's health and survival.

Chemical dependency does not occur in an isolated and impervious compartment of life. There is always some interaction between substance use and the surrounding people and circumstances. Rare are the chemically dependent nurses who do not have other serious issues complicating their life. Sometimes concerns are weighing heavily on the nurse regarding a loved one's health or a spouse's job prospects. There may be relationship, financial or legal difficulties which are present to some extent.

Some of these variables may be directly or indirectly connected to the nurse's substance use. In some instances, these other factors may not have been caused by the nurse's chemical dependency. However, even in these cases, any other existing issues have been further complicated by the nurse's drug or alcohol use.

Regardless of any possible association between chemical dependency and other current life situations, time away from nursing practice fosters and solidifies the nurse's belief that staying clean and sober must take precedence over all other matters. Because a leave from employment is such a hardship for most, it drives home the fact that the ongoing maintenance of recovery from chemical dependency must remain a top priority. This includes work, family, financial and other obligations. When all is said and done, if relationships, economics, professional duties or any other commitments come before treatment and recovery efforts, life itself is jeopardized.

Nurses who experience a reprieve from practice as a direct result of chemical dependency see the stark reality with crisp clarity: that without continuous, uninterrupted recovery from chemical dependency, there is no profession, no livelihood, no fiscal soundness, and no physical or emotional health. In a way, chemical dependency is the most predatory of lenders, worse than any corrupt mortgage broker or loan shark. The vulture with its hook in the chemically dependent nurse begins the collection proceedings much more abruptly than most borrowers are accustomed. The demand for payment very quickly boils down to "Your money or your life." But, ultimately, regardless of any arrangements for repayment, this lender makes a swift swoop to grab both.

The fallacy of placing any issue before recovery from chemical dependency is readily evident to nurses in other situations related to health. If the diagnosis was a heart attack, signing out against medical advice to tend to job duties would be seen as short-sighted and lacking sound judgment. No nurse would propose a substitute for the most expert care that a center of excellence could provide. Diluting treatment to what could be rendered on a haphazard basis to accommodate returning to work would never be entertained, as any shortcuts may very well cause death or disability. All other matters, job related or not, would be placed on hold.

The necessity for optimal, state-of-the-art treatment is no less important for a nurse with a chemical dependency. Continuing to work without any pause from practice during the initial stage of recovery does not usually offer the best outcome. When nurses are leveraged into ceasing professional endeavors for a time, there is a corresponding decrease in distractions that drain the nurse's time, focus and stamina. Work and other activities of daily life do compete with the time, attention and energy requirements of a fledgling recovery. These precious resources must be used judiciously, in order to accommodate the rigors recovery demands.

With one less pair of capable hands available for duty, employers may certainly feel challenged to adequately deliver health services to patients. However, any nurse who is actively using substances, or in a less than optimal state of recovery, is just a sentinel event away from harm to self and/or others.

Nurses in stable and ongoing recoveries, however, are usually excellent providers of care. Recovery efforts require nurses to develop enhanced coping skills and a better support network than they previously possessed. Frequently, recovering nurses have a keener sense of commitment and loyalty to their employer, colleagues and patients, as well as the profession. Usually there is a greater appreciation for what was nearly lost, barely salvageable and difficult to reclaim.

The efforts which recovery dictates, and that a reprieve from practice upholds, have an effect similar to physical exercise. Muscles of determination and perseverance have become hardened by disciplined conditioning, while the armor of invulnerability has become softened. The nurse's view of the world is adjusted, taking into account the needs of self and others. Reality is now essentially intact, no longer adjusted by the use of mood-altering chemicals.

Chemically dependent nurses in a solid and uninterrupted recovery are of immense value to employers, patients and the profession. They are well worth the patience and support which may be required to return them to practice. Similar to other serious conditions which may warrant a leave of absence, however, there are some customs which may enhance re-entry into the workplace. Some elements may assist in the maintenance of a continuous recovery. The following chapter focuses on programs which have been established in many states to assist in meeting this challenge.

Alternative To Discipline Programs

In the U.S., each state has enacted laws which may differ from neighboring states. Even within a state, municipalities may have the right to regulate certain activities within their borders. Distinct jurisdictions may impose codes defining expected versus unacceptable behavior. Rules mandating the recycling of paper and plastic, restricting the use of hand-held devices while driving, or forbidding smoking in public places may fall under the jurisdiction of local government.

When it comes to a driver's license, however, permission to operate a motor vehicle is granted at the state level. Usually this is obtained from the state of residence, although one may choose to hold additional licenses in other states. While valid licensure from one state is honored throughout the country, all drivers are held accountable for abiding by the laws of every area they drive through.

Like driving, the practice of nursing is a privilege granted at the state level. Individual states set the specific educational and clinical requirements individuals must meet in order to sit for the state licensing exam. Passing scores for these tests, as well as the definition of the scope of permissible practice, are also established by the state. The criteria necessary for license re-registration is also within the purview of the given state to determine. So, similar to permission to drive, the authorization to practice nursing is signified by a license bestowed by state government.

However, unlike our authorization to drive a motor vehicle, the privilege to practice nursing does not extend across any state lines. Valid licensure must also be obtained in any other state we wish to practice in. So, while nurses may have one driver's license to drive throughout the country as they please, additional professional nursing licenses are required if a nurse wishes to work in another state. Moreover, nurses are expected to fully conform to all the regulations within any state they practice.

States also set the standards for professional conduct, as well as the manner in which any complaints against a nurse will be investigated. Findings of any breach in the state's Nurse Practice Act or the state's definition of professional conduct, may lead to disciplinary action against the nurse. Professional behavior which is prosecuted in one state may very well be handled differently in neighboring states.

These distinctions between state laws governing nursing practice are noteworthy considerations, especially when looking closely at chemical dependency in the profession. At the time of this publication, alternative to discipline programs exist in about forty of the fifty states in the U.S. These programs were specifically created to handle some professional discipline issues in a non-punitive manner. They have been established because they often afford earlier identification of issues affecting practice and, therefore, more timely intervention, which can increase public safety.

Nurses who comply fully with the mandates of alternative to discipline programs are usually granted some immunity from professional charges which would normally be filed. The criteria for enrollment in such programs are determined by the state and not all nurses may qualify for admission. However, many nurses with chemical dependency issues do enter these programs.

Alternative to discipline programs are not treatment programs for chemical dependency. They do, however, often facilitate, encourage and sometimes require the nurse to undergo formal evaluation and subsequent treatment. While they generally yield to the recommendation of chemical dependency treatment providers who are rendering care, alternative to discipline programs may place additional stipulations on the nurse to meet the state's established requirements.

In states where these programs are available, such mandatory specifications usually include a minimum length of participation after acceptance into the alternative to discipline program. Multiple requirements for completion are set and must be met, which are determined by the state. While some specifics in one state's program may be somewhat similar to other states, there are often numerous differences. Significant distinctions, as well as subtle nuances which exist between states, can be mind-boggling. If one were inclined to do justice to any comparison between even a few states' alternative to discipline programs, an entire book on the subject would need to be written.

However, for the purpose of this publication, several key provisions which are found in most of the existing programs will be discussed. These common denominators will serve to illustrate some of the customary methods which have been used effectively in returning chemically dependent nurses to practice. For anyone who may wish to examine a given state in detail, an inquiry to the State Board of Nursing in a particular state may be helpful.

The very first allegiance of all alternative to discipline programs is safeguarding the public. These programs also value the nurse's professional contribution and seek to preserve the nurse's career, if the nurse remains substance-free. Thus, these entities aim at providing mandatory procedures which offer the best assurance of this goal.

Alternative to discipline programs should not be confused with any of the 12-step programs available, although participation in 12-step fellowships is very often strongly encouraged. One of the hallmarks of 12-step programs is their tradition of anonymity and practice of the twelve steps and twelve traditions, as outlined many decades ago by Alcoholics Anonymous.

Since it began, Alcoholics Anonymous has had no authority over its members, but it strongly discourages members from identifying themselves as members of A.A. in any form of public media. Attendance is on a strictly voluntary basis, without enforcement of any rules. There are no lists for verifying the attendance of members. Anyone who says they meet the membership requirement, which is a sincere desire to stop drinking, is a member. While some may hold service positions to ensure meetings run smoothly and some may be respected as members of longstanding with decades of sobriety, there is no hierarchy in the fellowship.

Other 12-step programs have arisen in response to problems other than alcohol. These other 12-step fellowships generally use the same basic twelve steps and twelve traditions as the foundation of their own program, although the focus and membership requirement will differ. Thus, in Narcotics Anonymous, or N.A., the powerlessness refers to drugs, instead of alcohol, and the person refers to themselves as a drug addict, rather than an alcoholic.

In contrast to 12-step programs, alternative to discipline programs are not at all anonymous. Though there may very well be some level of confidentiality present in alternative to discipline programs, the nurse is surely identifiable. There is not only the use of full name, but state nursing license number. Additionally, specifics related to a sentinel event or other professional documentation may be on file from the employer or another source. Past licensure applications and renewal forms, as well as other records, may also be readily accessible.

Also, unlike 12-step fellowships, the nurse is held strictly accountable for meeting any and all established requirements of the alternative to discipline program. While, technically, a nurse's participation may be categorized as voluntary, there is usually no absence of leverage. In fact, nurses may feel quite a bit of pressure exerted on them to enter an alternative to discipline program. Some of this duress may come from the State Board of Nursing or a disciplinary arm of the state's professional licensing agency. There may well be the threat of professional misconduct or other proceedings.

Thus, the nurse may be informed that charges will be forthcoming if the nurse does not enroll in the alternative to discipline program. An employer, in some instances, may mandate the entry and successful completion of all the alternative to discipline program's requirements as a condition of return to work and/or continued employment. If an alternative to discipline program is an option for a nurse, usually any demand for entry and ongoing compliance with its requirements is of great benefit to the chemically dependent nurse.

Another tradition of 12-step programs is that there are no specific admission criteria beyond a mere statement that one has a problem with a certain substance or behavior. However, an alternative to discipline program often requires any prospective participants to furnish an evaluation from a chemical dependency treatment provider. This must usually be accompanied by the specific diagnosis rendered by the specialist providing treatment. In cases where there may be a concomitant psychiatric or medical condition, there may be the need for additional documentation related to those issues.

Prior to enrolling the nurse, an alternative to discipline program may ask for evidence which confirms no harm befell any patients due to the nurse's actions. If a nurse has diluted, substituted or withheld medication from a patient, he or she might be precluded from participation in the alternative to discipline program as these situations are often considered injurious to patients.

The duration of enrollment in these programs varies. Most states demand a minimum of five years, over which time a nurse is monitored in their practice setting. Currently, the shortest minimum requirement of oversight a nurse receives in any alternative to discipline program consists of at least two years of monitoring after a return to practice. Some states initially established a two year minimum, but subsequently increased the period of monitoring to address a significant number of relapses evident in participants shortly after they reached the two year mark.

Depending on the circumstances, some states may permit re-entry to the alternative to discipline program if there is a subsequent relapse after successfully completing the program. However, professional discipline charges may be filed, and second chances are not necessarily granted in every instance.

States with alternative to discipline programs set monitoring standards which customarily include ongoing drug screening. The frequency and method of screening may vary according to the state, as well as the nurse's specific case. The goal of monitoring is to ensure that the nurse remains substance-free. Documentation with toxicology screens which are regularly reviewed offers this assurance.

Testing is usually required on a random basis, which may be set by the alternative to discipline program or the chemical dependency treatment provider. A random screening schedule means that the frequency of collection is not known by the nurse beforehand and varies from week to week. Thus, each day affords an equal opportunity that the nurse will be asked for a sample. Such an arbitrary schedule reminds the nurse of the ongoing requirement of abstinence from all mood-altering substances.

Usually urine and/or breathalyzer samples are collected. The frequency of testing may initially be more than once a week and later weaned down to several times a month. The number of times a nurse is tested is established by the alternative to discipline and/or the treatment provider.

Samples collected must usually be observed by a third party, who is responsible for verifying that the specimen was given by a particular nurse and that the sample was not tampered with. The term chain of custody regarding specimen collection denotes that certain strict protocols were followed to ensure the integrity of the sample. Thus, there is some verification that the specimen was not diluted, substituted or in any way manipulated by the nurse giving the specimen or the collector accepting the sample.

Nurses are often required to surrender their license to practice nursing as a stipulation to their enrollment in the alternative to discipline program. The length of time a nurse must be substance-free, prior to permission to return to practice, is usually several months. Although license restoration is determined by the alternative to discipline program, input is often solicited from chemical dependency treatment providers and other sources.

After return to work, an alternative to discipline program continues to monitor the status of the recovering nurse. Ongoing random and observed toxicology testing continues throughout the time the nurse remains in the program. Updated information regarding the nurse's ongoing status is usually obtained on a regular basis from treatment providers until the nurse is discharged from formal chemical dependency treatment.

Often an individual who has the ability to observe the recovering nurse regularly in their workplace is selected. Sometimes referred to as the worksite monitor, this individual furnishes updates to the alternative to discipline program. This information usually includes the nurse's appearance and behavior on the job. Attendance, punctuality, job performance and compliance with any practice restrictions may be included in these reports. This documentation provides some assurance that the nurse is acting in a manner consistent with recovery, as well as the state's established requirements regarding limitations on the nurse's professional practice. Periodically, these details are reviewed by the alternative program. At times, this may be done in conjunction with a face-to-face interview with the recovering nurse.

When the nurse returns to work, restrictions are usually placed on the nurse's license to practice. Some of these may be predetermined by the alternative to discipline program according to established customs. At other times, there may be additional limitations which are placed on the nurse due to his or her individual circumstances. Often, any recommendations from the treatment provider or worksite monitor are taken into consideration, although determinations are ultimately at the discretion of the alternative to discipline program. Some restrictions may be initiated based on the substances previously used, the area of clinical practice engaged in, or another factor related to the nurse's history or current situation.

Upon the initial restitution of the license and return to work, the nurse will usually be precluded from working in high risk areas. These are settings where there is frequent need to access and handle controlled substances. These areas may often include critical care, oncology, recovery room and emergency departments. Also, areas where a nurse has inconsistent or minimal supervision may be off-limits, such as homecare, private practice, agency, or float pool positions. Working nights is normally prohibited, as there is often less presence of supervision to provide oversight and less nurses available to accommodate any requisite practice restrictions. Additionally, night-shift work may adversely affect sleep habits, making a nurse in early recovery more vulnerable to relapse.

Travel or contract nursing, in which a nurse will have consecutive contracts of a few weeks' or months' duration, is often forbidden. Often these positions are in geographic regions or clinical areas which have a critical nursing shortage. Work arrangements such as these can appeal to nurses who wish to fly under the radar screen of detection. Such situations can decrease the chance that drug diversion is detected. Thus, these assignments can attract chemically dependent nurses because there is frequent rotation of new staff. Often, it takes time for suspicious patterns of behavior to become evident. Some facilities have decreased the likelihood that such an event will occur by drafting policies which deny access of all controlled substances to any nurse who is not a regular employee.

Alternative to discipline programs also usually restrict a nurse from working overtime, or more than forty hours per week. Individual cases may be taken into account, with some nurses only permitted to initially return to work on a part-time basis. As the recovery process demands much energy and time, alternative to discipline programs and treatment providers usually disapprove of any work in excess of full-time employment.

Some states have established mandatory peer support group meetings for the chemically dependent nurse engaged in the alternative to discipline program. Other states may offer optional peer support group arrangements. Some states may even allow chemically dependent nurses to take part in peer support groups when they are not enrolled in the alternative to discipline program.

Peer support group meetings may be overseen by agencies or individuals who are distinct and separate from the alternative to discipline program. In such cases, a certain amount of feedback may be provided to the alternative to discipline program. Any details furnished will be added to the ongoing information from treatment providers and the workplace to determine the nurse's ongoing recovery status.

One of the underlying rationales for offering peer support group meetings which can only be accessed by recovering nurses, is that these forums offer a place where ongoing issues unique to the nursing profession can be aired freely. Nurses are extremely ashamed of their behaviors related to chemical dependency. These groups afford a level of acceptance, identification and trust that promotes bonding, which is often absent from groups open to any chemically dependent person. Taboo and shameful topics related to drug diversion may be discussed candidly which promotes further healing and recovery. Supportive relationships with recovering colleagues are fostered. Pertinent dialogues regarding return to practice are shared. Fears regarding a recovering nurse's return to a former employer, or the search for new employment, are often discussed in detail. Trust grows with the passage of time, while the struggles, accomplishments and hopes of recovery are expressed and validated.

This ability to fully disclose any past or present troubling incidents, without fear of ridicule, ostracism or retaliation by non-nurses is extremely helpful to the nurse's recovery process. Without an avenue to safely bring to light any and all circumstances related to chemical dependency, nurses may disavow, soft soap or forget the past. This may lead to a repetition of history, which in the recovering nurse's case would equate to a return to substance use.

With full disclosure, nurses find understanding recovering colleagues, who lend their support and encouragement. The importance of this, however, is not just essential for the purpose of uplifting morale. These groups also offer some of the most essential ingredients required for effective confrontation. Telltale warning signs of impending relapse, which may not be recognized by a recovering nurse, rarely escape the attention of a whole room full of recovering colleagues.

For many nurses who have become fully integrated into a peer support group, there is no better place for such a confrontation to occur. Recovering peers can identify troubling attitudes and/or behaviors and interpret them precisely. There is no one who knows the terrain better than those who have taken the same detour, yet exemplify an ongoing recovery.

Thus, words of supportive encouragement, as well as direct confrontation, resonate freely on a wavelength which is transmitted with laser-like precision. Often, nothing comes nearly as close to the well-timed strike by a recovering colleague, which frequently leaves no room for side-stepping or denial.

Peer support groups are not available in every area, and attendance requirements vary between states. Some alternative to discipline programs mandate a certain level of participation, with only a handful of excused absences permitted per year. In some programs, going below the requisite level of participation in peer support group meetings prompts notification to the State Board of Nursing that the nurse is non-compliant with alternative to discipline standards.

Although 12-step attendance may be strongly encouraged at a certain frequency per week, due to anonymity in A.A. and N.A., this may be difficult to verify. As most alternative to discipline programs meet in-person with the nurse periodically in order to assess their status, such interactions may include specifics related to the nurse's 12-step participation. Many alternative to discipline program personnel are quite astute in their ability to extract information and intonation which identifies any embellishment of 12-step involvement.

Enrollment in the alternative to discipline program carries no cost in some states, other than the fees associated with toxicology screens and formal treatment. In some instances, the funds to provide alternative to discipline program services are collected by means of a surcharge paid by every nurse licensed in the state, regardless of whether such assistance is ever required. In other states, nurses pay a monthly premium for the duration of their enrollment in the program. An additional fee may be set for each peer support group meeting attended.

As a nurse progresses in recovery, the restrictions originally placed on nursing practice are gradually lifted. Some recovering nurses do decide, of their own volition, to refrain from certain scopes of practice, even after they are permitted to engage in unrestricted practice. While many recovering nurses do return to full duties safely, without difficulty, others opt to practice within one or more self-imposed practice restrictions.

One of the most frequent limits a nurse in recovery may select, even after completion of an alternative to discipline program, is only working in a position where there is minimal or no access to controlled substances. For nurses who have diverted drugs, this is sometimes a wise choice.

Other nurses may opt to remain off the night-shift, particularly if that interfered with sleep patterns. In some cases, nurses have decided to refrain from high stress areas of practice or positions which entail an inordinate number of hours to work each week.

For chemically dependent nurses who have completed an alternative to discipline program and plan to relocate, consideration should be given to the impact such a change will have on licensure. Because most states handle chemical dependency in the profession differently, a nurse may be required to meet additional criteria, in spite of having met all of the previous state's mandates. Therefore, thorough research into such a matter should be conducted by any nurses who have had an issue with chemical dependency or been enrolled in an alternative to discipline program.

Those who practice nursing in states where there is no alternative to discipline program may have no recourse available which mitigates any professional charges filed. However, over the past decade, many states have established alternative to discipline programs. Whether the remaining states will join the ranks of the eighty percent who have developed such initiatives remains to be seen.

That alternative to discipline programs safeguard the public, while sparing nurses from professional misconduct charges and fostering their recovery, is unequivocally true. But return to practice in an uninterrupted state of recovery entails much more than any state mandate. There is an ongoing need for vigilance on the part of the recovering nurse. There are many factors which can support or undermine that focus. The following chapters look more closely at the challenges nurses, colleagues and employers face when bringing a nurse back to work.

Return To Practice

On occasions when the nurse entered recovery prior to an issue being evident in the workplace, the commencement of work after recovery may simply be a matter of providing medical clearance to resume work. Examples of this may be a nurse who is convicted of driving while intoxicated and leveraged into recovery as a result.

However, in many cases, an issue with chemical dependency has been identified by an employer or a regulatory agency. In situations like these, several months may pass before the nurse re-enters the workforce. Most often, the timing for such a resumption of practice is not solely up to the nurse. Frequently, treatment providers, alternative to discipline programs, employee assistance programs and/or other parties may have a role in the decision-making process.

While agreement between all parties regarding when the nurse is capable of returning to work may be preferable, if an alternative to discipline program is involved, authorization to engage in practice is ultimately at the state's discretion. While many recovering nurses may object strenuously to what they often view as an unnecessary delay, such protests are not likely to hasten their return to work.

Each scenario is quite unique, given the complex variables of each state's requirements and the specifics related to an individual nurse's particular situation. Complicating the matter further are the details surrounding the professional setting in which the nurse returns to practice. Naturally, any restrictions imposed on the nurse's license are significant variables which need to be addressed. Additionally any monitoring requirements stipulated by an alternative to discipline program must be taken into account.

Sometimes when an employer is aware of an issue with chemical dependency, the nurse is afforded the opportunity to return to the facility. However, in some cases the nurse is terminated from employment. Such dismissals may occur when the nurse is initially confronted, or after there is a close investigation into the nurse's actions. At other times, the nurse may have required a lengthy leave of absence for treatment which the employer was unable or unwilling to honor.

Although recovering nurses seeking a new job have many obstacles to overcome, nurses returning to practice in their previous settings have their own challenges. In instances where a nurse is able to return to their former employer, considerations include effective strategies which safeguard and support return to practice and continued recovery. If the state has an alternative to discipline program in place, the protocols established certainly offer safety precautions for the nurse and the public. However, some facilities may have developed additional policies which exceed those safeguards and better meet the specific needs of the organization. Thus, some of these employers have formulated practices based on former experiences with recovering nurses returning to work.

For instance, while an alternative to discipline program may prohibit the nurse from administering controlled substances, they usually allow the nurse to administer other drugs, such as antibiotics, diabetic and cardiac medications. However, employers may make an administrative decision that the recovering nurse will not be permitted to pass any medications whatsoever. In lieu of not performing any medication-related duties, the nurse may be assigned other skilled nursing tasks, such as wound care, or starting and maintaining intravenous lines.

Beyond the scope of alternative to discipline programs is the challenge that employers face in effectively handling a wide array of potent emotions and attitudes from co-workers regarding the recovering nurse's return to work. As much as an organization may have respected and protected the nurse's right to confidentiality after a sentinel event, people do have a tendency to talk. News may travel, regardless of attempts at containment. Colleagues are not blind to the absence of the nurse, nor are they likely to be totally oblivious to investigations into a nurse's actions. Even when documentation is inspected quietly by supervisors to ascertain whether discrepancies exist, it is often natural for staff to speculate, making assumptions which may or may not be correct.

The undercurrent of feelings and attitudes about the entire situation is usually quite palpable, in spite of an employer's efforts to smooth the way for a nurse's return to work. The reactions among co-workers may run the gamut, either openly or secretly, beneath the surface. That responses can be quite unpredictable is an understatement.

Those on the periphery of the incident may accept the nurse back without batting an eye. Others not formerly fond of the nurse may be receptive to the recovering nurse's return to the fold. After all, the arrival of the skilled hands of one familiar with the institution's policies and procedures is a godsend to any unit. However, those closest to the nurse may at times experience the most conflict. Welcoming the nurse back with open arms may be more difficult for those closest in proximity, as well as affection. There may very well be feelings of betrayal and mistrust. For any individuals who may have unresolved issues of their own or a family member related to chemical dependency, there may be lukewarm aloofness or scorching contempt.

Meanwhile, the recovering nurse, who is about to return to a former workplace, has his or her own mixed feelings. Typically, there is a deep sense of gratitude for receiving a second chance. Most nurses returning to their former job realize that many of their recovering colleagues were not so fortunate to receive such an opportunity. The recognition that they have been taken back, therefore, is not usually taken lightly.

There is quite an assortment of other thoughts and feelings, however, which may serve as a compost of very strong emotions. Some of the chief among these are shame, fear and anxiety. For the most part, the recovering nurse experiences much anguish over past behavior related to substance use. Fear and anxiety often abound in anticipation of returning to work. Some of these feelings are

163

natural trepidation over the reception from colleagues. Uneasiness may also revolve around one's ability to perform job functions which now must be conducted within certain mandated parameters. Performance anxiety may be in attendance, particularly if the leave of absence was prolonged. At times, nurses may even begin to question whether they have forgotten clinical skills which had been second nature just a few months earlier. While the recovering nurse's identity as a licensed professional remains largely intact, some may actually wonder whether they really know how to be a nurse without the use of substances.

Unquestionably, employers deal with a nurse's return to practice in a variety of ways. The amount of attention or publicity the nurse's past behavior or leave of absence may have received might be one consideration. Established methods of dealing with similar situations in the past may have determined a model for effectively handling these situations. However, some past experiences with returning recovering nurses to practice may have yielded less-than-optimal outcomes. The past relapse of a nurse may have indicated a need for the fine-tuning of procedures. Certainly, what works in one facility may not be possible, practical or even advisable in another setting.

Determinations regarding policies may require ongoing tailoring, as circumstances arise, and as experience dictates. For this reason, some employers may take a multidisciplinary team approach, in order to spearhead the evolution of protocols based on lessons learned. Members of such focal groups may include representatives from human resources, administration, legal department, pharmacy, employee health, collective bargaining and/or the employee assistance program. As it is difficult for personnel inside an organization to objectively analyze the issue in its entirety, an impassionate third party may be consulted. At times, this combination of in-house personnel with one or more unbiased experts may assist an institution in the development of initiatives which eliminate any existing deficiencies in procedures.

Sometimes, facilities may use a nurse's return to practice as a timely occasion for a presentation on the subject of chemical dependency in the profession. This may be provided by staff-based educators, employee assistance program personnel or an addiction specialist. Some institutions may wish to highlight information for everyone in the organization. Other employers may choose to offer a smaller, more intimate venue, available only to the specific unit the recovering nurse is rejoining. In many cases, the recovering nurse will meet with key members of management to discuss details, prior to such a forum being held. In this way, any concerns or questions which the employer and/or the nurse have may be discussed privately, beforehand. Thus, both parties may reach a better understanding of each other's position, as well as an accord.

In some instances, the recovering nurse may be invited to a unit-based staff meeting prior to his or her return to duty. This may serve as an excellent time for the nurse to become re-acquainted with colleagues, before taking on the added demands of a work assignment. This more relaxed and often less distracting environment may permit the recovering nurse to express any apologies he or she may wish to extend to co-workers. Thus, the shroud of what has been left unspoken is lifted and feelings regarding the past situation may be defused to some extent.

Whether this occurs somewhat openly in a group setting or privately, in one-to-one exchanges with select peers, depends on an infinite number of variables. That there is an opportunity available for such discussion to take place is often helpful in reducing tensions for all concerned. Often, when this is done in some manner, the subject may no longer be perceived as an unspeakable albatross, where thoughts run rampant without expression, taking on a life of their own.

Some situations, however, may be better handled without any group forum of discussion. In a large institution, particularly when the nurse is to be reassigned to a totally new area, a departmental airing may be inappropriate. This may be a case where the only person needing any information about the recovering nurse is the supervisor who makes the schedule and duty assignments. This need-to-know may largely be determined based on whether any of the recovering nurse's customary tasks include ones which are forbidden by the alternative to discipline program. In such a situation, the communication of at least some specifics may be warranted to ensure that all mandates are enforced.

For the recovering nurse who is cleared to return to work, but has no former employer to return to, the hurdles are somewhat different. While there may be no worries about the reception from colleagues or any need for the expression of remorse, the nurse does face the difficult challenge of finding a new position which corresponds with a limited scope of practice.

Unbecoming A Nurse

Finding an employer willing to accept any necessary accommodations can be an arduous task. The proper job fit is critical, however, and often more complex than locating a position which allows the nurse to remain within any state imposed limitations. A facility's willingness to cooperate with what is being required of the nurse is indispensable.

Therefore, the recovering nurse's selection process includes intangible qualities, such as an atmosphere of support or understanding from the prospective employer. During a job interview, key personnel often communicate the organization's culture, as well as attitude, either directly or subtly. The impression given by superiors in the organization, especially any individuals the nurse would directly report to, is of critical importance.

In obtaining a new employer, most nurses are usually best served if they take whatever period of time is necessary to find the closest possible match. Jumping into a less-than-ideal position should be avoided, in spite of the temptation to seize the very first job that comes along. Often being out of the workforce for several months tends to cause one to become impatient with their quest for a job. This tendency, however, must be tempered with thoughtful consideration that a less-than-optimal fit

168

may prompt the need for another change in job, in very short order. Therefore, if a prospective employer does not or cannot offer the recovering nurse optimal safeguards, as well as a supportive atmosphere, it is usually far better for the recovering nurse to pass on the opportunity.

Additional factors to weigh are the time and travel requirements of any job. As nurses in alternative to discipline programs are required to give toxicology samples regularly and with very little notice, any employment obtained will need to be readily accessible to where screens must be collected.

The proximity of the worksite to the chemical dependency treatment provider is also a factor, as many nurses continue these services after return to practice. Because changing treatment sites can be very disruptive to the nurse and create possible gaps in the documentation provided to the alternative to discipline program, many nurses use every means possible to remain engaged in treatment with their original provider.

The location of the 12-step meetings one has been attending regularly is another variable to contemplate. While consistency and familiarity with these groups are important, there is frequently an abundance of these meetings to choose from. It is likely that there will be far fewer options of nurse peer support group meetings available as they are relatively new compared to 12-step meetings. Additionally, as they sometimes require state funding, there are apt to be far fewer in existence, in spite of any growing demand. Thus, while 12-step and peer support group meetings are both very important assets in a recovering nurse's arsenal of supports going forward, there may be far less latitude in switching some of these meetings.

Every nurse who has established sufficient recovery milestones to return to practice must use ongoing care and discretion in selecting future employment settings. The hallmark of any recovery from chemical dependency is a protective and supportive network of individuals who should be asked for guidance and input in times of indecision. There is no better time to perfect this positive recovery trait than when one is exploring prospective employers and job settings. Nurses in recovery who discuss circumstances such as these with their sponsors, treatment providers and/or other confidantes, prior to stepping back into their nursing shoes and scrubs, exemplify a strong model of recovery.

While most nurses view return to work as a right-of-passage which indicates good progress in their recovery, there is a need for ongoing vigilance. Recovery from chemical dependency is similar to other chronic, potentially fatal conditions. There is a continuous need to partake in the activities which fostered recovery in the first place. Also, there is an ongoing requirement to recognize and disarm any thoughts, attitudes or behaviors which may lead one towards relapse.

The next chapter addresses some of the warning signs which recovering nurses and those closest to them may discern from time to time. As chemical dependency has often burned the recovering nurse severely, and the recovery process has exacted much in the way of time, expense, energy and commitment, most nurses wholeheartedly want to avoid any proximity to the flames of relapse. Remaining as distant as possible from any circumstances or behaviors which may ignite a return to substance use is, therefore, essential for these nurses.

Warning Signs Of Relapse

Many naturally assume that after experiencing an imminent threat to one's health, career, or life, one would steer clear of any activity possibly leading to subsequent difficulty. Especially when future repercussions may likely include even more serious outcomes, many may believe that such a person would always take the very safest course of action possible. However logical this train of thought is, it is an incomplete depiction of the situation involving anyone with the disease of chemical dependency.

If one were diagnosed with chronic kidney failure, one would likely undergo dialysis a few times each week, for several hours per session. The aim of this treatment would be to remove accumulated waste products from the bloodstream, which are customarily excreted by healthy kidneys. Many patients would opt to comply with this treatment, if recommended by their doctor.

Other instructions accompanying such a diagnosis would likely include extensive dietary restrictions. Most patients would attempt to follow such advice, at least to some degree. While some may veer off their food plan from time to time, most would continue to attend their dialysis appointments, precisely as ordered, because the treatment makes them feel better.

The importance of adhering to treatment has probably been discussed in no-nonsense terms by the patient's kidney specialist. This, coupled with the experience of well-being which dialysis provides, further motivates the patient to comply with instructions. While it is unlikely that any patient finds the ongoing regimen enjoyable, most are grateful that such treatment exists, because it gives them the ability to continue much of their normal activities.

The nurse with a chemical dependency also has a chronic, potentially life-threatening disease. Whatever precipitates the nurse's entry into treatment, usually astute awareness of the stark reality of the situation is not far behind. At this point, many nurses may be eager to bring about a remedy, in order to get their family and professional life back in order. Usually chemical dependency treatment educates the nurse regarding the chronic, progressive and permanent nature of the condition. The need for continued care and ever-present vigilance, in order to keep the disease in remission, is usually underscored repeatedly. The nurse often begins attending 12-step meetings, such as Alcoholics Anonymous and/or Narcotics

Anonymous, and continues through the earliest phase of treatment.

Exposure to other chemically dependent individuals who succumb to a relapse is likely to occur while attending 12-step meetings and/or treatment groups during this period. Observing the experience of relapsing individuals dramatically highlights the ongoing hazard which any resumption of use holds for the nurse. Treatment continues, progress is made, and the recovering nurse begins to feel hopeful. While reminders of the negative consequences to profession, finances and relationships are unmistakably present, milestones in recovery are achieved. Maybe the nurse is about to regain professional licensure, or has already done so. The nurse may be about to return to their former work setting or begin an entirely new job. The trust of family and colleagues may be a bit shaky, but improving somewhat.

Things may be going fairly well, or even extremely well, in light of past events. Yet, the nurse may relapse. This is a mind-boggling, seeming contradiction to everyone, especially the nurse. Many wonder aloud, as well as to themselves in the privacy of their own thoughts and hearts, what happened? The nurse is as flummoxed as the spouse, parents, children, colleagues, friends and employer. With so very, very much at stake, how could this happen to a bright, educated and now treated nurse?

Upon closer inspection, this phenomenon may be better understood, though it maintains a certain mystifying and troubling quality; for unlike chronic kidney failure, in which the difficulty resides in the kidney, the seat of chemical dependency is lodged in the brain. Although hands may tremor, pupils may dilate or constrict, speech may slur, gait may wobble and sweat may be profuse, all these symptoms are initiated by the effect of one or more substances on the brain. This organ is the central location where all thought processes and self-regulatory mechanisms reside. This serves as the switchboard, so to speak, which moderates all behavior. The ability to think rationally, as well as rationalize one's thoughts and actions, occurs here.

The brain is the hub from which information is relayed to all other parts of the body, producing involuntary as well as volitional processes and movements. Breathing is maintained, heartbeat is regulated and blinking is initiated. Much of the brain's functions take place without conscious thought. Even with deliberate intent, any attempts to override the brain's automatic processes are

175

usually well beyond our conscious ability to control.

One of the brain's chief tasks is to maintain homeostasis. This is the baseline state our body perceives as the status quo of health. The brain goes about doing everything within its power to maintain this delicate balance. Thus, the brain will automatically and simultaneously perform a wide variety of regulatory actions to achieve this goal. In this way, body temperature is kept constant, fluid balance is maintained and oxygen levels remain sufficient to meet the demands of exertion.

The brain, however, is the organ most vulnerable to substance use. The term mood-altering substance was coined because of the powerful affect these chemicals have on the brain and the resultant change in feelings experienced after their ingestion. Likewise, the phrase habit-forming came about in response to the pleasurable sensations which entice one to continue the use of these substances.

Neurotransmitters which carry information from one nerve cell in the brain to another are altered by chemical use. Once changed, the previous state of homeostasis is compromised. The delicate balance of the brain is now essentially different from the baseline state prior to the introduction of mood-altering substances. Therefore, the chemically dependent brain is significantly different from the brain of the non-chemically dependent individual. The changes in the brain due to drug use are widely believed to persist permanently, without any return to the previous, pre-chemical dependency state.

The brain's knack for sparking memories which may unconsciously trigger cues from the environment is also highly significant. While little consideration may be given to this ability of the brain in most situations, it is a key element involved in the phenomenon of craving which is experienced by many chemically dependent individuals. Thus, environmental cuing can occur without any conscious awareness. In this way, certain sights, sounds, smells, feelings, people or activities, which have been unconsciously linked with past chemical use, may prompt memories which are accompanied by cravings.

The desire for the effect produced by one or more substances may not be immediately followed by a conscious thought to reinitiate use. In fact, the recovering nurse may be unaware of any overt urges to use. Logical thoughts based on past experience with negative outcomes may slip the nurse's mind. The brain's phenomenal ability to rationalize may take precedence, initiating either a straightforward or convoluted process which abruptly or circuitously leads back to drug and/or alcohol use.

This irrational mental twist observed in chemical dependency circles has long been referred to as the cunning, baffling and powerful attributes of the disease. These three adjectives underscore, quite accurately, that intelligence, in tandem with a highly sophisticated ability to rationalize, may actually be a liability to individuals in recovery. Thus, for some, there may be an almost trance-like acquiescence, rather than a protective, defiant stance just prior to relapse. Operating by rote, the brain, which has been habituated to the effect of mood-altering chemicals, may set in motion a chain of imperceptible thoughts which lead one to procure and use substances.

The phenomenon of craving may not be fully eradicated, although it may be dampened or managed effectively with a combination of strategies. Most of the time, chemical dependency treatment programs will outline very specific recommendations for a nurse, based on individual needs. While most nurses will be urged to attend 12-step or other self-help programs, some may be prescribed medications to alleviate cravings and/or block the effect of substances.

Whether or not such a medication is prescribed, the mindset of the recovering nurse is still susceptible. In spite of how well the nurse may feel or what treatment milestones may have been met, the achievement of an uninterrupted recovery from chemical dependency requires ongoing vigilance and sustained effort.

Relapse is most effectively prevented by taking daily actions which support and enhance the awareness of one's continued vulnerability. Of equal importance is the belief that the prospects of an ongoing recovery are very good when there is continued compliance with activities which initiated recovery.

The occurrence of relapse, although often not consciously evident to the nurse, is often highly predictable. Frequently, warning signs are readily apparent to those closest to the recovering nurse. While relapses, like individuals, may differ somewhat under the closest scrutiny, there are some typically characteristic markers indicative of a nurse backsliding into trouble. Some signals may be more subtle, while some are definitely easy to overlook; but all of the following should be cause for heightened concern.

Some warning signs fall into the category of attitudes which telegraph increased risk, such as the recovering nurse who refers to their history of substance use or a sentinel event as something that is behind them. Phrases such as "that won't happen ever again," or "I know I won't do that again because I'd lose my license" depict this demeanor. Expressions which give voice to the belief that one is safely beyond repeating substance use because they have been enlightened by the experience of detrimental consequences are noteworthy. When verbiage infers an attitude of invulnerability the recovering nurse is often headed for difficulty. Feelings equated with being enlightened or impervious to relapse truly scream loudly to others of an elevated risk of impending relapse.

The attitude that one has graduated to safer ground, based on a number of months or years in recovery, is also a possible signal of trouble ahead. This is a most ominous sign when a nurse is skipping some or all of the fundamental requisites of 12-step participation. This is referred to as "talking the walk", rather than "walking the walk." Nurses who decrease or totally break contact with their sponsor, decrease or halt their 12-step meeting attendance, slack off or never initiate 12-step activities are putting their recovery in a precarious state.   Instances   when   communication   with recovering peers is shrugged off, either insidiously or abruptly, are especially dangerous.

Additional signs of an approaching storm are the re-initiation of behaviors which accompanied or precipitated prior substance use. The nurse who used to work seventy hours each week prior to recovery, and then returns to that demanding schedule, may very well be inviting trouble. If depression was a factor which precipitated the use of substances to improve one's mood, any recurrence of depressive symptoms should be taken seriously and prompt formal re-evaluation. Likewise, the nurse who worked nights in a high stress position with minimal oversight and frequent access to narcotics may see an escalating need for release. If the stress cannot be effectively managed and continues to build without respite, substance use may be reinitiated.

While relapse may not occur for weeks, months or years, one or a combination of these factors are almost always detectable before the substance is used. As chemical dependency is progressive in its course, relapse is often more severe than the nurse's past experiences. Moreover, repercussions after a relapse often carry a corresponding greater consequence than was initially experienced.

Relapse is never a requirement for a full and uninterrupted recovery from any disease. This is equally true for the disease of chemical dependency. In fact, the avoidance of relapse is paramount, given that any additional use leads to more profound changes in the brain. If one recovers and never relapses, the habitual practice of positive behaviors which recovery demands become more ingrained and natural. Just as substance use took on a life of its own, so too does a recovery which is sustained over time. While the brain of the individual may never return to the pre-chemically dependent state, maintaining behaviors which support recovery will enhance future health and the achievement of a continuous, uninterrupted recovery.

While the recovering nurse faces an ongoing need to remain substance-free, there are many nurses who have made the requisite adjustments. While none would intentionally go out of their way to have acquired this condition in the first place, many are firmly convinced that their life in recovery is far better than their life was before it.

More than standing sentry, watching and waiting for the development of warning signs which may be identified too late, there is an ongoing need for continuous quality improvement in dealing with this challenge. The following chapter offers food for thought, proposing some strategies which may preempt problems in those yet to be identified as chemically dependent. Just as importantly, it may alert nursing students and prospective students to the need for self-care and self-survey of their own potential risk.

As most of these suggestions cannot possibly be initiated without the collective cooperation of several people from many different walks of life who are dedicated to preventing chemical dependency, these proposals may appear extremely lofty, if not nearly impossible.

However, for nurses who have died or come close to death, their families and friends, colleagues and treatment providers, as well as employers, there may be no greater cause which we could devote ourselves to. Whether a spark of disagreement is lit throughout the following pages, or thoughtful contemplation is ignited, either would be a long overdue tribute to all who have labored on this issue.

Preemptive Strategies

The quote at the beginning of this book was an excerpt from a statement made nearly a century ago by William D. Silkworth, M.D. He served as the medical director of one of the first hospitals in the United States which treated alcohol and drug addiction. His words typify the reality experienced by those living with and providing treatment to chemically dependent individuals. For most, this struggle and suffering reverberates to the core of their being. Certainly, there is no short supply of pain and tragedy in the world. But, as Helen Keller once noted, the world is also full of the overcoming of suffering.

For over two decades now, my thoughts and efforts have pivoted around the situation of chemically dependent individuals, and those interacting with them. For whatever reason, however, I find it even more distressing when dealing with the plight of the chemically dependent nurse. Granted, some of this concern may be rather self-serving, as one who will, undoubtedly, require the skilled and compassionate care of a nurse at some future time. Yet, more than that, having witnessed their immense heartache, as well as that of their relatives, friends, colleagues and employers, it is no wonder that this dilemma invades my sleeping moments, just as it did Dr. Silkworth's.

After giving this subject an inordinate amount of deliberation, to the point that it became an almost all-consuming preoccupation, I must present some preemptive approaches. To sit back, with the self-satisfaction that I may have helped some with their affliction, does absolutely nothing to appease my restlessness and dissatisfaction with the widely held statistic that at least one in ten of my peers will succumb to this condition. There is nothing I have seen which reflects that this trend is about to abate. In light of the prediction that there will be an even greater demand for licensed nurses over the next decade, this issue will most likely escalate, rather than decline, in significance.

I believe that the ultimate success of any strategies will require more than a simple outline of action steps to be taken. I am of the firm opinion that making proposals, prior to exploring the attitudes towards this issue, would be extremely short-sighted. Additionally, I believe it would be immensely disrespectful to those who have very legitimate and often intense feelings on this subject. Therefore, prior to broaching any specific suggestions, I will try to accurately portray some of the viewpoints I have heard from others, and have

185

personally held over my thirty-three years as a nurse.

My own thoughts and beliefs about nursing were originally woven of a silk which was first spun by my parents; then elementary and high school teachers; and, ultimately, our culture. This perspective became easily distinguished from my parents' and other layperson's views, as my professional training and experience as a nurse advanced. That some of these beliefs had their origin in fiction rather than fact, without close scrutiny to any preconceptions I may have had, is an understatement.

Faulty beliefs, once apparent to me, may have been a relatively simple matter to overcome, that quite naturally would prompt a change of mind. But it is another thing entirely to overturn emotions and attitudes sufficiently to persuade a change of heart. At least, this has been my experience, which became apparent to me in my attitude towards the chemically dependent patients I cared for when I floated to a detox unit in 1976.

The transparency of what I then saw as manipulative behavior, and an undisciplined lifestyle, was incompatible with the values I was raised with. I must confess, and am sorry to say, that I stood in judgment of these patients. At the time, the only evaluation I could make, based on the economy of my core beliefs and my upbringing, was that these individuals were "less than" or "weak-willed." While performing my professional duties, I was never in any way unkind, and all my patients received the best care. However, my attitudes certainly sprung from a hypercritical mind, which righteously stood in judgment of those afflicted with chemical dependency.

Of course, as I worked more closely with these patients, I absorbed new information, knowledge and understanding of their condition. As my attitude became enlightened, so did my heart. It was not very long before I found that the more I studied addiction, observed the behavior of those in its grasp, and interacted with them, the more my viewpoint changed. Prior righteous indignation evaporated with comprehension, which gave birth to a blossoming compassion for their plight.

In hindsight, though, I now see an even finer distinction, regarding my initial care of alcoholics in detox in 1976: it is the fine line between caring for patients, and caring about them. I am dismayed that this discernible difference, which never escaped my eye as a nine-year-old patient in the

1960's, was lost to me for several years as a new nurse. As a child, I was an astute observer, aware of the very obvious and fundamental difference between the nurse who gave me the enema and the nurse who spritzed me with perfume. While both were certainly qualified professionals on all counts, the one nurse lacked the radiant warmth, empathy and compassion of Kathleen, who made it crystal clear that she cared, not only for me, but about me. While caring for patients will do in a pinch, if my condition can ever withstand any delay, I'll wait for the nurse who cares about me, as well as for me. I'll wait for Kathleen, or one of her protégés.

But just because I became compassionate in my care for and about the chemically dependent patient, this did not necessarily equate to an empathy which went out across the board, to everyone. One of my deepest regrets is that a genuine compassion was not readily and wholeheartedly extended to nurses with this disease.

I, like many colleagues, had difficulty accepting those I worked with who had an issue with chemical dependency. This was especially true if their chemical dependency led to diversion of controlled substances. I too, on occasion, would whisper in hushed tones about the nurse being offered the option of resigning, in lieu of termination, for such actions.

One of my core beliefs, which did not undergo complete overhaul until the 1980's, was that, as nurses, we were educated and licensed. Therefore, we should be above acquiring a chemical dependency. I fully believed, at the time quite subconsciously, that because we "know better," we should "do better" and "be better."

As I later examined this philosophy, however, I was appalled to find it was rooted in an arrogance that we, as nurses, should know and do better because I thought, erroneously, that we were better. This warped thinking was based solely on the premise that because we had become nurses, we were somewhat a cut above others. This translated into us being capable of escaping at least some of the frailties of others. To this day, of course, I have never been able to locate the nursing text or lecture from which this position was affirmed.

Once I began to view nurses as ordinary, everyday people, undoubtedly with talents, skills and education, but just as prone to every condition, even chemical dependency, did my conceit subside. I started to see through and beyond what I had presumed was sheer weakness of character in a nurse. I commenced to perceive the chemically dependent nurse as I would any other chemically dependent person whom I had come to care for, and care about.

I am immensely grateful that this altered opinion, that nurses are people too, with strengths and foibles, came long before I began working exclusively with chemically dependent nurses. I shudder to think of the inadvertent fallout that such a belief would have had on the nurses I met. If one remnant of the notion had remained, that chemically dependent nurses were somehow responsible for having acquired this condition, an untold amount of damage could have been done. That the nurse was and is accountable for taking their chemical dependency seriously, and getting treatment, is absolutely true. Nurses also shoulder the total responsibility for vigilantly, persistently and consistently taking all the steps necessary to optimally ensure their recovery.

However, I have also come to believe that nurses are as blameless as anyone else for having this disease. Like the patient who has heart disease or diabetes, no chemically dependent individual is at fault. Just as I have yet to meet any patient who intentionally set themselves up to acquire heart disease or diabetes, so too have I yet to meet the chemically dependent nurse who went about deliberately flirting with the disease. In fact, in working with the chemically dependent nurses, it was nearly always apparent that they had made a most conscious effort to do quite the opposite. Clearly, in spite of this desire, a critical detour had been taken. This makes it all the more strikingly sad, as well as ironic, that the most genuine intention to do right went so wrong, missing the mark entirely.

The insights I gained from witnessing the struggles and successes of these nurses, however, placed me in the eye of the storm. From this unique and privileged position, I was safe and secure, able to be ever-observant of their ups and downs. Although aware of the high wind velocity and torrential rains experienced by the afflicted nurses, I began to realize that I could easily lose sight of where I had come from: the periphery of that storm, as experienced by the non-afflicted nurses who are in the vast majority. Thus, I began to identify a formidable challenge: to put myself back in the shoes of the floor nurse who was not as privy to the innermost circumstances of the chemically dependent nurse.

As I knew from my own initial prejudice as a nurse, my understanding of chemically dependent nurses was sparse. In order to effectively present this topic, I had to take into account all perspectives. To do that, I had to don my whites of long ago: the cap, the uniform, the shoes; as well as my prior beliefs, values and preconceptions. I needed to recapture the nurse I once was, when I graduated nursing school. I had to reacquaint myself with the nurse who walked long corridors and suctioned patients on respirators. I had to relive the necessity to step back from a patient's bedside, prior to defibrillation and then, just as quickly, lean in closer to check for a pulse.

I must place those same fingers, now not nearly as smooth, on the pulse of who I actually was, as a nurse at the bedside, where the majority of my peers remain. It became necessary to lace the shoes of my many colleagues, the roughly ninety percent who never had, and never will have an issue with chemical dependency. Those millions of nurses who have not, and hopefully will not, unbecome their profession, or themselves.

As the nurse at the bedside, and later the charge nurse, the actions committed and omitted by my colleagues were extremely important to me. We worked hand-in-glove, turning patients, getting them out of bed, covering each other for coffee and dinner breaks. We pitched in, when and where we were needed, for the good of the patient, the unit and the facility. We were part of a team.

As we became more seasoned in our professional setting, we felt a certain sense of entitlement, since seniority should, and often does, afford us certain perks. With longevity comes a better opportunity to have first dibs on Thanksgiving, Christmas and New Year's Eve holidays off. The prime weeks for vacation and better work assignments, with somewhat less use of brawn, were also anticipated with seniority. As our years and expertise advance, we generally expect to garner better salaries and more time off. We believe we should be the ones to get first crack at overtime work when desired, and the opportunity to decline it, if that should be our preference.

Therefore, it was only natural for me to feel a bit annoyed, frustrated and unappreciated for doing the right thing, when my less tenured colleague received an accommodation after diverting drugs from the unit. In fact, how could I not feel unacknowledged, dismissed and often somewhat victimized when that very same nurse may have jeopardized patients, as well as myself and my license? Certainly, counting the narcotics, accepting the shipment of controlled substances and witnessing another co-worker's waste is the role of the nurse, but the chemically dependent nurse initially returning to work is usually exempt from those tasks.

So, at times I felt slighted that I must remain at the bedside, while the nurse who just returned from a medical leave for chemical dependency treatment was provided with the temporary assignment reviewing charts, making follow-up calls, or triaging patients. Often there was the belief that I did everything, by the book, and this nurse did wrong. Why am I not getting my due, while this nurse is being catered to? Then, to add insult to injury, I continue to work the night shift, while this nurse gets the day slot which I applied for months ago. These are just a portion of the feelings and concerns that staff nurses have expressed to me, and that I have had myself.

Yet, when examining this issue from all the sides I have now been privy to, there is another equally potent perspective: that of the nurse in recovery. These nurses, although accommodated in their restrictions, are usually required to drop their pants, or raise their skirt, while someone observes them urinate into a specimen cup an enumerable amount of times over the course of two to five or more years. The cost of this may not be completely covered by insurance, if it is covered at all.

Formal outpatient treatment often continues, even after return to work, one or more times per week. If not covered by insurance, between this treatment and the urine drug screen costs, the recovering nurse is often on the financial hook for monthly payments which far exceed any lease on a brand-new luxury car.

Furthermore, attendance and full participation at Alcoholics and/or Narcotics Anonymous meetings are strongly encouraged several times a week. For nurses following the recommendations of most treatment providers and utilizing a very proactive and vigilant recovery approach, easily ten or more hours per week may be spent in attending treatment and 12-step meetings alone.

Though any professional discipline charges may be held in abeyance for those who have successfully completed their alternative to discipline program requirements, documentation regarding this matter is usually kept on file with the professional licensing agency indefinitely. This issue may be brought to the fore in the future, even in cases where the nurse has not relapsed. The cost of attorney representation may cost a few thousand dollars to defend any charges of professional misconduct. If criminal charges are ever filed, additional legal representation is often needed, and the expense escalates dramatically.

In addition to all this is the fact that the recovering nurse is usually out of work for several months. When this equates to loss of health benefits, coverage for chemical dependency and any other treatment evaporates, leaving the burden to the nurse or public assistance. In instances where the nurse carries these benefits for the entire family, the lapse is even more devastating.

Certainly, this is the first nurse investigated if there is any future discrepancy in medication records. Of course, any future relapse may pose permanent loss of nursing license and additional professional or criminal charges.

Florence Nightingale, who lived in the 1800's, has been attributed with elevating the profession of nursing from its less-than-admirable reputation. She is known for her tireless efforts caring for wounded soldiers in the Crimean War. Due to their experience with her, they aptly named her the "Lady with the Lamp." This moniker was derived from the beacon of light, which emanated from her oil lamp and surrounded her, as she made her rounds each night. It is from these roots that the oil lamp has become the symbol of the nursing profession.

Having read about Ms. Nightingale in 1973, I re-read parts of her story some thirty-three years later. It prompted me later to wonder if she would have ceased her nightly trek, turned her gaze, as well as her hands and lamp, away from anyone who required her support. I speculated whether she would have judged these maimed soldiers, and found them unworthy of her compassionate care if they had been driven to actions she disapproved of. Instead of weapons of war, if their afflictions had arisen from a stigmatized illness, like chemical dependency, would her mercy have run dry? Had these soldiers been caught in the crossfire of their own chemical dependency, rather than military engagement, would her attention and lamplight been extinguished? If the skirmishes had existed in their minds, rather than on the more prominent battlefield, would we have some other symbol today by which to signify our profession?

The issue of chemical dependency in the profession raises many complex questions, without ready-made solutions. As such, there may be few, if any, absolutes to offer. However, there is no doubt that this dilemma needs vastly more attention than it has received. This is especially true if we hope to adequately address concerns and initiate preemptive, rather than retrospective and reactive, strategies.

We live in a time when so much of what was unfathomable in my parents' generation is now taken for granted. This is an environment where technology intersects readily with our identification of needs. Thus, advances have been made in nearly everything, from replacing ailing hearts to constructing new limbs. The adage "where there is a will, there is a way" has become more than a figurative term. In this atmosphere, improvisations are born to meet many societal concerns.

One such issue which has benefitted from technological innovations was the warning system of Amber Alerts, which did not exist when I was growing up. These bulletins have been met with much public support, for few would refuse to render their assistance in reuniting a child with their parents. Yet, with all due respect for the magnitude of the problem of child abduction, at least one in ten nurses has been or will be abducted by chemical dependency in their lifetime. As there is no sign that this phenomenon is abating, and a steep rise in our need for licensed nurses over the next decade is predicted, this statistic is even more alarming.

A prerequisite to all change, especially when tackling complicated issues, is the suspension, at least in one's mind, of the status quo or the heretofore preferential method of doing things. In spite of living in an imperfect world, I am in complete agreement with Robert Browning's sentiment that "A man's reach should exceed his grasp - or what's a heaven for?"

While I may have no ability on my own beyond writing this book to effect a change for the better, I will outline some suggestions which may be helpful, and which hopefully others can improve upon. These proposals may be well received by some or deemed insufficient, extreme or even useless by others. Regardless of their reception, however, one of the necessary steps seems clear: that interest must be sparked to a sufficient magnitude that it will not be snuffed out easily.

As this book, once published, is no longer a living document which can be amended, I have taken great care in exercising good judgment in my use of words and phrases. Any tendency I may innately have as an individual to be extremely forthright and outspoken verbally has, therefore, been tempered with due thought and deliberation throughout this work. I have great respect and appreciation for the challenges and difficulties policymakers, educators, employers and regulatory agencies face in dealing with the complicated facets of this issue. However, in situations where my professional experience has unequivocally shown that harm has, indeed, already come to some, my use of discretionary language has ethically yielded, where necessary, to words which communicate greater candor. We are, after all, dealing with life and death matters, not just of a few nurses and an untold number of patients, but an unmistakable amount of human pain and suffering.

In spite of the bulging curriculum which exists currently in nursing schools, there is a dire need to place this topic at the very top of the list. This subject is of such enormity that its rightful place belongs at the threshold of the educational process. I hold this opinion because of the many years I spent consulting to various businesses on occupational health and safety. Those entities which were most successful, as well as profitable, have been those which incorporated and consistently fostered the most fundamental of policies: safety first.

Therefore, in the interests of student welfare, and that of the public, this matter should ideally be introduced as part of the orientation process, before students even begin their initial classes. Similar to other inherent occupational risks, this subject should be highlighted repeatedly, throughout the educational process, providing a rock-solid footing for student nurses.

Because of the nature of chemical dependency, students should be enticed by incentives or, possibly, obliged by mandates, to bring one or more relatives or friends to receive vital information about the risk of chemical dependency in the profession. While knowledge certainly offers no blanket of immunity, there is no reason for a cloak of ignorance to persist. Loved ones need to be educated, for they are in an ideal position to objectively gauge a change in affect or behavior on the part of the nurse. They are the student's cornerstone of support, and as such, deserve and need this information.

That relatives and friends may not always be able to assemble the pieces of the chemical dependency puzzle with total accuracy should not deter us from providing vital specifics, which may assist them with spotting early indications of a possible issue. After all, preventing a problem in the workplace is of utmost concern to the nurse, their loved ones and society.

Continuous education of all nurses must become as frequent and as commonplace as recertification of our CPR skills. Obviously, the ninety percent of nurses not affected by chemical dependency are in the proximity of those who are affected. Detection of warning signs, and knowing, by rote, exactly what to do and what not to do is as significant here, as it is in the case of a fire.

As early identification is key, the conduction of self-survey on the part of every nurse is warranted. Implementing this practice on a personal basis is, in itself, another early detection tactic, like self breast exams. Though neither will ever replace the value of a professional evaluation, both do keep one attuned to the potential of a problem, and afford one the opportunity to act accordingly.

Employers need to be forthcoming, on a regular basis, reporting any and all suspicions of drug diversion or deterioration in a nurse's status, as per applicable laws. It is doubtful that any who hire nurses to any great extent have totally escaped engaging a chemically dependent nurse at their facility. If any have been able to do just that, they may have best practices which should be shared with other employers in their industry. However, it seems more likely that some organizations may have turned a blind eye to more or less evident indications of an issue.

Regulatory agencies with jurisdiction over drug enforcement and matters of public welfare are numerous. For those entrusted to oversee nurses in their professional practice or for ensuring that controlled substances traverse a direct course from manufacturer through to the legitimate, intended recipient, the challenges are indeed very great. While there have definitely been watchful eyes on this predicament within the profession, it would appear that a total absence of reported suspicions from any institution employing a large number of nurses should be questioned.

Undoubtedly, in times of financial crisis, such as we face today, agencies and individuals may have greater limitations on what they can reasonably be expected to accomplish. In spite of this, it seems there must be some method in a computerized age of tracking facilities of longstanding existence which have always employed vast numbers of nurses administering controlled substances. For any of these which have yet to file even one single report of a suspicion of diversion, a closer look seems justified.

In this way, institutions would be advised that a statistically unlikely absence of reports would be cause for closer scrutiny. Thus, employers may be leveraged into more consistent, proactive and humane conduct toward chemical dependency in the profession; for I am of the enduring conviction that to discharge any nurse suspected of drug diversion from employment, without the requisite notification, offers the potentially inhumane outcome of death to the nurse, as well as danger to patients.

Great strides have been made in protecting the public and restoring the recovering nurse to practice in states with alternative to discipline programs. The distinctions between states which have these programs are extensive, and research needs to be conducted to determine the level of effectiveness of each different approach used.

The absence of alternative to discipline programs in approximately twenty percent of the states in the U.S. is of concern. It begs the question of whether chemically dependent nurses, who have not displayed any depraved indifference to patients, are summarily rounded up and housed in jails, at public expense. In an era of unprecedented financial woes, in which recovery from chemical dependency is an uninterrupted reality for many, this situation, if it exists, seems a poor use of tax dollars.

With all due respect to prosecutors, who may rightly believe that the chemically dependent nurse owes a debt to society, the absence of harm to others should be taken into account. In such cases, if sentence is indeed to be levied, it appears that drug court and/or community service may be a more viable and cost effective option. In a time when there is overwhelming demand in society, surely there is a more useful purpose these nurses can offer, without endangering public welfare. Surely, these nurses could be mandated to provide blood pressure screening to senior citizens in a library on a weekly basis or some other function which offers no risk to the public.

That chemical dependency is so baffling and misunderstood is an understatement. Like severe depression, which may lead one to attempt or actually take one's life, those afflicted with chemical dependency are powerless to rid themselves of their malady. As much as it would be an injustice to throw the book at each depressed individual who tries to commit suicide, it seems just as ill-advised to respond to chemically dependent nurses in a similar manner.

However, having said that, there are a small number of nurses who display attitudes and behaviors which are inconsistent with recovery. A rare few give a clear indication that they have an attitude of entitlement, which qualifies them to conduct themselves as they please, regardless of the danger to others. In my experience, these nurses have numbered less than a dozen out of the several hundred chemically dependent nurses I have interviewed and interacted with professionally since 2003. This limited group of individuals, like all chemically dependent nurses, remains blameless for having this disease. Nevertheless, they do require special handling which adequately ensures the public safety. Therefore, the interests of society may dictate that the few who have unequivocally demonstrated depraved indifference to patients be precluded from returning to the profession.

As recruitment campaigns throughout many geographic areas are underway to attract individuals to the profession, it seems reasonably prudent that measures should be taken to present the potential risk for prospective nurses. There are possible perils associated with every livelihood and the presence of occupational hazard does not usually dissuade one who would be an otherwise good match for any profession.

If the ultimate goal of enticing men and women to become nurses is to meet the demand for this highly educated and skilled profession, it appears wise to outline any potential for risk, early in the process. Without the utmost concern for those potentially selecting this career path, the ultimate fulfillment of the role may become interrupted for some, possibly short-circuiting a career, as well as a life. As this bodes poorly for meeting recruitment, as well as safety needs, the utmost attention should be given to this matter.

A world with better safeguards, where a nurse's risk of chemical dependency is diminished, is a worthwhile goal, in spite of any challenges. Nurses have a right to receive adequate and full support as they fulfill their professional duties in the manner in which Ms. Nightingale and my nurse, Kathleen, did. However, such a world will only be possible with increased awareness of the risk, acceptance of the situation as it is today, and consistent efforts directed at optimal improvement.

I hope that recovering nurses will come together, in tight-knit clusters, offering support to one another. Individually and collectively, you are the ones most capable of facilitating an about-face for a colleague headed for the brink of relapse. Often in the best position to see the trap of chemical dependency for what it is, you also have the ideal frame of reference from which to speak candidly with another nurse. Most frequently, it is your recognition of the imminent signs of relapse which is impeccably accurate. It is also your timely response to any such telltale threats which can be best tolerated, as well as heeded by your colleague.

Not a soul is responsible for actions taken or refrained from by others, including relapse. Feigned ignorance to the slippery path a fellow recovering nurse is traversing may seem like the easier, softer way when compared with a loving confrontation. But that comfort may be short lived if at least one solid attempt at a candid discussion is not initiated before a relapse occurs. Shielding any nurse from your awareness of warning flags seems, at least to this nurse, very much like allowing a patient to pull out a life-sustaining tube.

Hopefully, this book can reach scores more than I could ever have touched personally. The possibility that a nurse's parent, child, administrator, educator or spouse can be spared, prior to a sentinel event, is my fondest desire. Although some of you may have a perspective different than mine, hopefully we will all strive, in our own ways, to discover common ground, as well as remedies which offer optimal safeguards for all.

I do know that there is hope for all chemically dependent nurses, even after having experienced a sentinel event. Absolutely, beyond all doubt, there is cause for much hope. But when my own hope seems to ebb with the weight of this dilemma and the lives adversely affected, I often pause to reflect on one utterly astonishing phenomenon that has never failed to buoy my continued efforts.

Less than a century ago, about one hundred of the lowest, most disdained, gutter level alcoholics wrote a book. They were, by their own admission, some of the most egotistical and self-centered people ever born. Conceivably, they could not utter even two consecutively coherent words when drunk. Yet, they managed to sober up, work collectively, and co-author a brilliant publication, outlining a blueprint of recovery for alcoholics.

That program has grown to a worldwide fellowship of great renown, which has grandfathered many other fellowships for people with still other problems. Although nearly a century later, this is the same world. And in a world like that, anything, absolutely anything, is possible.

List of Resources

Al-Anon Family Groups (Al-Anon) is an international fellowship that has only one purpose - to help families and friends of alcoholics. They do this by practicing the Twelve Steps of A.A. themselves, encouraging and understanding their alcoholic relatives, and welcoming and giving comfort to families of alcoholics.
http://www.al-anon.alateen.org or (757) 563-1600

Alcoholics Anonymous (AA) is an international fellowship of individuals who share their experience, strength and hope that they may recover from alcoholism.
http://www.aa.org or (212) 870-3400

The American Association of Nurse Anesthetists (AANA), the professional association for Certified Registered Nurse Anesthetists (CRNAs) and student nurse anesthetists, has offered expertise in peer assistance for 25 years. The website provides excellent information on chemical dependency in the profession, and links to valuable resources which nurses outside the specialty may find helpful.
http://www.aana.com or (847) 692-7050

American Nurses Association (ANA) is the only full-service professional organization representing the nation's 2.9 million registered nurses (RNs) through its 54 constituent member associations.
http://www.NursingWorld.org or (800) 274-4262

Center for Substance Abuse Treatment (CSAT) is a federal agency which is under the Substance Abuse and Mental Health Services Administration (SAMHSA). The website is helpful in identifying chemical dependency treatment.
http://www.findtreatment.samsha.gov or (800) 662-HELP

List of Resources

The International Nurses Society on Addictions (IntNSA) is a professional specialty organization for nurses with a mission to advance excellence in addictions nursing practice through advocacy, collaboration, education, research and policy development.
http://www.intnsa.org or (877) 646-8672

Narcotics Anonymous (NA) is an international fellowship of individuals recovering from drug addiction, who practice the Twelve Steps and Twelve Traditions of N.A.
http://www.na.org or (818) 773-9999

Nar-Anon Family Groups (Nar-Anon) is a worldwide fellowship for those affected by someone's addiction. As a Twelve Step program, they offer help by sharing their experience, strength and hope.
http://www.nar-anon.org or (310) 534-8188

National Suicide Prevention Lifeline offers support to those in crises and can be accessed via internet or phone.
http://www.suicidepreventionlifeline.org or (800) 273-TALK

Professional Health Program Resource Network assists professionals in finding recovery services.
http://www.phprn.com

The Robert Wood Johnson Foundation (RWJF) is the nation's largest philanthropy. The Foundation is devoted to improving the health and health care of all Americans by working with a diverse group of organizations and individuals to identify solutions and achieve meaningful and timely change. Their website offers much information on chemical dependency.
http://www.rwjf.org or (877) 843-7953

Substance Abuse and Mental Health Services Administration (SAMHSA) is a federal agency focused on facilitating recovery in people who have, or are at risk from, mental or substance use disorders. http://www.samhsa.org

Suggested Reading and Viewing

Addiction, The HBO Series. Produced by John Hoffman and Susan Froemke. DVD is available through www.hbo.com. Home Box Office, 2007

Al-Anon and Al-Anon Family Group Headquarters. *Paths to Recovery – Al-Anon's Steps, Traditions and Concepts.* Virginia Beach, VA: Al-Anon Family Group headquarters, Inc., 1997.

Alcoholics Anonymous World Services, Inc. *Alcoholics Anonymous.* New York City, NY: Alcoholics Anonymous World Services, Inc., 1939, 1955, 1976, 2001.

Conyers, Beverly. *Addict in the Family: Stories of Loss, Hope and Recovery.* Center City, MN: Hazelden Publishing and Educational Services, 2003.

Hoffman, John and Susan Froemke, eds. HBO's *Addiction: Why Can't They Just Stop?* New York: Rodale Press, 2007.

Johnson, Vernon. *Intervention: How to Help Someone Who Doesn't Want to Be Helped.* Center City, MN: Hazelden Publishing, 1986.

Mooney, Al J., Arlene Eisenberg and Howard Eisenberg. *The Recovery Handbook.* New York, NY: Workman Publishing, 1992.

Moyers on Addiction: Close to Home. Directed by Bill Moyers. VHS. Curriculum Media Group, 1998.

Moyers, William C., and Katherine Ketcham. *Broken: My Story of Addiction and Redemption.* New York: Viking, 2006.

The SHUNT Self-Survey For Nurses™ Scoring Sheet
Copyright © 2008 Paula Davies Scimeca   All Rights Reserved
www.unbecominganurse.org email: paula@unbecominganurse.org

No score indicates a total absence of risk, nor any certainty that anyone is, or ever will become, chemically dependent.

YES = 1 NO = 0

S - Social withdrawal or self-isolative behavior.   ____

S - Self-care behaviors beneath societal, professional
    or the nurse's own standards.   ____

H - History of chemical dependency in the nurse's
    immediate family.   ____

H - History of negative consequences related
    to the nurse's substance use.   ____

U - Untreated or unremitting emotional or physical pain. ____

U - Using medication for a reason it was not intended
    or in a manner not recommended.   ____

N - Nursing practice routinely in excess of
    55 hours per week.   ____

N - Nursing duties include frequent access to
    controlled substances.   ____

T - Transitional period requiring major adjustment
    within the past year.   ____

T - Turmoil or tragedy with unresolved conflict.   ____

DATE:_____   TOTAL= ____

213

A message from the author

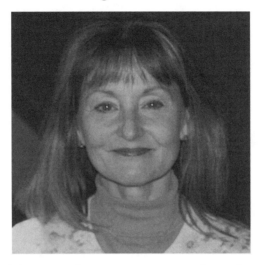

One of the most frequent comments from those who reviewed the manuscript prior to publication was the hope that there would be the addition of anecdotal summaries of actual nurses throughout the book. While I am certain the inclusion of such narratives would have added depth for the reader, it may have compromised the confidentiality of those I have worked with over the years.

For those of you who may wish to share your personal experience, strength and hope as a recovering nurse in a future volume, please feel free to email me at paula@unbecominganurse.org. As loved ones witness the devastation described in these pages firsthand, they have equally poignant accounts to offer. I would gladly do my part to ensure that your voice is also heard.

Regards, Paula

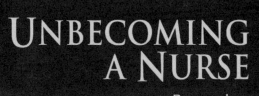

UNBECOMING
A NURSE
Bypassing
the Hidden
Chemical
Dependency
Trap

Paula Davies Scimeca, RN, MS

To order copies please visit our website:
www.unbecominganurse.org
or write us at:
Sea Meca, Inc.
PO Box 090455
Staten Island, NY 10309